28 days to Younger skin

28 days to Younger skin

The diet program for beautiful skin including more than 50 recipes

Karen Fischer

Robert
ROSE

For complete cataloguing information, see page 244.

Disclaimer

This book is a general guide only and should never be a substitute for the skill, knowledge, and experience of a qualified medical professional dealing with the facts, circumstances, and symptoms of a particular case.

The nutritional, medical, and health information presented in this book is based on the research, training, and professional experience of the author, and is true and complete to the best of her knowledge. However, this book is intended only as an informative guide for those wishing to know more about health, nutrition, and medicine; it is not intended to replace or countermand the advice given by the reader's personal physician. Because each person and situation is unique, the author and the publisher urge the reader to check with a qualified health-care professional before using any procedure where there is a question as to its appropriateness. A physician should be consulted before beginning any exercise program. The author and the publisher are not responsible for any adverse effects or consequences resulting from the use of the information in this book. It is the responsibility of the reader to consult a physician or other qualified health-care professional regarding his or her personal care.

This book contains references to products that may not be available everywhere. The intent of the information provided is to be helpful; however, there is no guarantee of results associated with the information provided. Use of brand names is for educational purposes only and does not imply endorsement.

The recipes in this book have been carefully tested by our kitchen and our tasters. To the best of our knowledge, they are safe and nutritious for ordinary use and users. For those people with food or other allergies, or who have special food requirements or health issues, please read the suggested contents of each recipe carefully and determine whether or not they may create a problem for you. All recipes are used at the risk of the consumer. We cannot be responsible for any hazards, loss, or damage that may occur as a result of any recipe use. For those with special needs, allergies, requirements, or health problems, in the event of any doubt, please contact your medical adviser prior to the use of any recipe.

Caution: Before beginning the Younger Skin Diet, be sure to consult a medical doctor or a dermatologist. If you have medical conditions that are being treated with diet or drugs, follow the Younger Skin Diet with the supervision of your doctor or dietitian.

Design and Production: Daniella Zanchetta/PageWave Graphics Inc.
Editors: Bob Hilderley, Senior Editor, Health; and Sue Sumeraj, Recipes
Copyeditor: Kelly Jones
Proofreader: Sheila Wawanash
Indexer: Gillian Watts

The publisher gratefully acknowledges the financial support of our publishing program by the Government of Canada through the Canada Book Fund.

Published by Robert Rose Inc.
120 Eglinton Ave East, Suite 800
Toronto, Ontario   M4P 1E2
Tel. (416) 322-6552 Fax: (416) 322-6936
www.robertrose.ca

Printed and bound in Canada

1 2 3 4 5 6 7 8 9 FP 22 21 20 19 18 17 16 15 14

Contents

Introduction

● ●

"You can be gorgeous at 30, charming at 40, and irresistible for the rest of your life."

— Coco Chanel

Fountain of Youth

According to legend, the Spanish explorer Juan Ponce de León first heard of the Fountain of Youth when he sailed to Puerto Rico in 1506 or 1508. Ponce de León had settled in Hispaniola, and his slaves built a grand house for him. But he was depressed. The years he had spent at sea battling harsh weather conditions had wrinkled his skin like an old apple, and the decades of drinking wine had swelled his belly. Then one day, according to legend, he overheard one of his Indian slaves say, "In Bimini no one grows old."

"Bimini! What is Bimini?" he asked.

"It is a beautiful island fragrant with flowers that lies far to the north of us. There is a spring of clear water and everyone that bathes in it becomes as young and strong as he was in his best days."

Ponce de León asked around. This fountain seemed to be common knowledge among the slaves. He made up his mind to conquer Bimini and claim the Fountain of Youth as his own. Ponce de León prepared three ships. In 1513, after exploring several islands to no avail, the Spaniards discovered a strange coast where the land was covered with flowers. It happened to be Easter Sunday, or Pascua Florida, which means "the Feast of Flowers," so Ponce de León named the land Florida. The Spaniards also found bountiful lemon and orange trees in Florida, and they collected their seeds.

Ponce de León roamed the land, drinking from clear springs and bathing in many streams and lakes, but he did not regain his youth, and he eventually gave up the search. Ponce de León returned to Florida in 1521 to establish a Spanish colony, but the natives fought back, and Ponce de León was struck by an arrow. "Take me back to Spain," he wailed, "for I shall never find the Fountain of Youth." His ship carried him to Cuba, but he soon died from his wound.

Ponce de León's search for a miraculous spring may have been fruitless, but he did discover a remarkable remedy for scurvy in the lemons and oranges his soldiers and sailors ate in Florida. These fruits could heal the skin and extend life expectancy. This was so revolutionary that it would take the rest of the world more than 200 years to discover this cure.

> Ponce de León's search for a miraculous spring may have been fruitless, but he did discover a remarkable remedy for scurvy in the lemons and oranges his soldiers and sailors ate in Florida.

Suffered by sailors and land-dwellers alike, scurvy was, at the time, a baffling disease where your skin slowly fell apart due to lack of vitamin C in the diet. The first signs were dry skin and mysterious bruising, fatigue, and cracked and bleeding lips. As the vitamin C deficiency worsened, the skin would become bumpy, and old wounds reopened as the skin's collagen bonds weakened. Sufferers eventually bled to death. In fact, in 1595, a Dutch fleet sailed to the East Indies with 249 men, and they returned 2 years later with only 88 survivors because they did not eat enough vitamin C–rich fruits and vegetables.

In 1747, more than 200 years after Ponce de León, British surgeon James Lind was credited with discovering the cure for scurvy. It took another 100 years for citrus fruits to be accepted as a legitimate treatment. In 1932, vitamin C was isolated as the therapeutic nutrient in treating scurvy, and although vitamin C was not the Fountain of Youth originally sought by the Spanish explorer, it was one piece of the anti-aging puzzle.

Searching for Younger Skin

The desire to have skin that shows no sign of aging is universal and transcends time. The ancient Egyptians had many rituals for beautifying themselves. Cleopatra, the Queen of Egypt, bathed in sour milk, which was rich in skin-smoothing lactic acid, and women in ancient Rome rubbed their skin with fermented grape skins (resveratrol-rich remnants from the bottom of wine barrels). Ancient Chinese emperors sent sailors in search of youth-restoring pearls. Today we have Botox, lasers, and fillers (to name a few) to magically smooth our skin.

I believe everyone has the right to do whatever they like in the quest for beautiful skin, so I am not going to admonish anyone for using artificial options. We are so lucky to live in an era where many anti-aging treatments — both natural and artificial — are available if we wish to use them. However, many of us are still searching for that miracle quick fix — a Fountain of Youth — that will make us young again. But we are overlooking one major fact: your skin is made from the foods you eat. According to several research studies, many North Americans still suffer from scurvy because people are simply not eating enough fruits and vegetables. It's a simple reminder to include healthy food in your beauty regimen.

Mirror, Mirror…

According to U.K. researchers from the Centre for Appearance Research (CAR), 90% of women don't like the way they look. There are women who also dread looking in the mirror, with 39% saying it brings up negative feelings about themselves. There is even a movement in the United States where women are avoiding mirrors. Mirror fasting — where people cover up all the mirrors in their house and avoid their reflection — is not the answer to low self-esteem and it can promote unhealthy self-neglect in some cases.

Your appearance — your weight, your skin, your waistline — gives you valuable clues about how healthy you are on the inside, so it is important to look at yourself for an honest appraisal once in a while. For example, if you have prematurely aged skin, it could indicate you are eating too many AGEs — advanced glycation end products — in your diet. Some simple changes could lead to younger-looking skin and potentially increase your lifespan. Sagging skin or poor skin tone can indicate you have a deficiency in the mineral copper. A large waist size can predict a risk of diabetes and heart disease. Being unhappy about your waistline can prompt you to change your diet, which could one day save your life. Loving who you are begins with being honest about what you like and dislike, caring about your feelings (even the bad ones), and then cheering yourself up by taking loving care of yourself.

I wish someone had told me to look after my skin and eat healthy food when I was younger. I spent some of my childhood in Darwin, Australia, in a town where it was always hot and sunny (except during cyclone season, when it rained). My nose constantly peeled from playing in the sun, and my diet was an unhealthy combination of strawberry milkshakes, toast, and pies (oh, and I loved french fries and chocolate mousse). I never considered eating a salad. No surprise that my first wrinkle appeared by the time I was 18. I remember thinking I looked so old!

> Some simple changes could lead to younger-looking skin and potentially increase your lifespan.

As I grew up, I have wanted one thing above all others — beautiful skin. It is one of the reasons I became a nutritionist. Since my teenage years, I have suffered from many skin complaints, including blemishes on my face and severe dermatitis on my hands. At one stage, psoriasis covered half my body. I used cortisone cream on my face for many years, which thinned my skin. I was always getting ill and I felt tired all the time. I thought there was something seriously wrong with me. I kept asking my doctor to run tests, which always came back looking okay, and each time, he would prescribe healthy food and exercise for my ailments. I'm a little bit stubborn and I need scientific proof before I will even consider changing my habits, so I read hundreds of research papers on skin health while I studied nutrition and completed a health science degree. This took more than 4 years (I told you I'm stubborn), but I'm glad I did.

Since changing my diet, I no longer suffer from skin disorders, but my quest for younger skin has intensified. Researching and writing this book has been a great joy.

Why 28 Days?

28 *Days to Younger Skin* is a fast-track program designed for people who have a special occasion coming up, such as a wedding or holiday, or any event at which you want to look your best. It can be used to complement your current beauty regimen, or if you are having a cosmetic procedure, you can use this program to supply the nutrients in your diet needed to speed up your recovery and enhance your results.

It is a 28-day program because it takes that long for your body to produce new skin cells in the deeper skin layers and for them to travel to the surface of your skin — so it is literally the beginning of a new you by Day 28. In addition, the program includes 28 menu plans, with recipes for a month of meals. It also takes about 21 days to form new habits, so by the end of the program, you might automatically continue with some of your new healthy habits.

The program is designed to boost your metabolism and supply all the nutrients needed for skin repair, renewal, and maintenance. It can also improve your energy and feelings of well-being, making it healthy for your whole body. There's also plenty of non-diet information to make choosing the right anti-aging skin care a breeze.

The 28-day program can improve the following conditions:

- Premature aging
- Fine lines and wrinkles
- Dry skin
- Rough or bumpy skin
- Poor skin tone and cellulite
- Mild age spots and hyperpigmentation
- Excessive body odor and bad breath
- Fatigue and sluggishness
- Hypoglycemia (food-related)
- Inability to lose weight
- Abdominal bloating
- Poor immunity to colds and flu
- *Candida albicans* infestations
- Slow wound healing
- Poor exercise recovery

Inner Health

Beauty is not only skin deep — if you look after your skin, you will improve your inner health, too. More than 200 million people worldwide suffer from osteoporosis, and in women over 45 years of age, brittle bones account for more days spent in hospital than many other diseases, including diabetes, heart disease, and breast cancer. However, if you look after your skin, you improve your chances of living without one of these conditions. The program in this book can also be used to lower your cholesterol levels and control blood sugar to decrease your risk of type 2 diabetes.

Because everyone is unique and you probably have specific desires when it comes to improving your skin, this program can be tailored to suit your needs. For example, if you have stubborn conditions, such as cellulite, dry skin, or acne, you can look up the specific course of action provided in the quick reference guide at the front of the book. Keep in mind that 28 days is a very short period of time and this program is designed to work fast, so be prepared — you will have to do some work every day during the 28-day period. But it will be worth it, and you can enjoy younger skin at the end of the program.

> Beautiful skin enhances people's lives and promotes self-confidence. At the end of this program, you will be able to look in the mirror and feel comfortable in your skin.

Beautiful skin enhances people's lives and promotes self-confidence. At the end of this program, you will be able to look in the mirror and feel comfortable in your skin. Self-confidence is one of the most attractive features you can possess. Enjoy the program. I wish you good health and happiness on your way to younger skin.

Quick Guide to Skin Problems and Their Treatments

Here is a convenient list of common skin problems, their causes, and their cures. Preview this list now and read on to gain a better understanding of your particular condition. Make notes in the margins, and come back to this list whenever you need a reminder.

Skin problem	Treatments	Referrals
Abscesses, skin ulcers, bacterial skin infections		See your medical doctor
Acne	Follow the 28-day program: avoid fried foods, red meat, dairy, sugar, almonds, flax seeds, and cooking oils; change skin-care products (they could be causing the problem); drink 8 glasses of filtered water daily; drink fresh vegetable juice; check for zinc or vitamin A deficiency; use anti-scar silicon sheets over healing acne to prevent scarring	For supplement advice, speak to a naturopathic doctor or read the acne chapter in *The Healthy Skin Diet*
Aged skin	Follow the 28-day program: wear a hat and sunscreen (at least SPF 30 on the body and SPF 50 on your face, neck, chest, and hands); take a calcium and omega-3 supplement	A cosmetic physician or dermatologist can advise on other options
Age spots (liver spots, sun spots, lentigines) on sun-exposed areas	Use pigmentation fade/bleach creams; use AHA skin-care products; wear SPF 50 sunscreen, especially on hands, face, and chest, to limit new ones from appearing (SPF 30 or less is not enough to prevent age spots)	A cosmetic physician or dermatologist can advise on stronger treatment options, such as laser treatment
Bruising, easy or with no apparent reason; purplish spots on skin	Check for vitamin C deficiency (early scurvy sign)	See your medical doctor
Bumpy skin or keratosis	Follow the 28-day program: take an omega-3 fish oil supplement or flaxseed oil daily; avoid cigarette smoke; check for vitamin A, zinc, or essential fatty acid deficiency	See your medical or naturopathic doctor if symptoms persist
Cellulite	Follow the 28-day program: avoid dairy and alcohol; drink filtered water daily; do toning exercises and soft-sand jogging; take a calcium supplement	

Skin problem	Treatments	Referrals
Chest wrinkles after sleep	Avoid drinking alcohol; apply body butter to area before and after sleep; use AHAs and retinol in skin care; sleep flat on your back; drink 8 glasses of filtered water daily; wear SPF 50 sunscreen if exposing your décolletage to the sun	
Dandruff	Follow the 28-day program: change your shampoo (avoid SLS/sulfates in shampoo); try this recipe for tea tree shampoo: add to your shampoo 1 tsp (5 mL) apple cider vinegar and ½ tsp (2 mL) tea tree oil, and shake (shampoo daily until symptoms improve)	Take a probiotic supplement (containing *Lactobacillus rhamnosus*, *L. rhamnosus GG*, and/ or *L. acidophilus LA-5*)
Dermatitis or contact dermatitis	Avoid contact irritants and refer to *The Eczema Diet* for dietary and skin-care advice	
Dry skin	Follow the 28-day program: take a calcium supplement; drink 8 glasses of filtered water daily; take an omega-3 fish oil supplement or flaxseed oil daily; use almonds and rice bran oil in cooking; avoid vitamin A supplements because they dry the skin; eat guava, papaya, and other yellow foods; use suitable moisturizers	
Eczema	Refer to *The Eczema Diet* for dietary and skin-care advice	
Enlarged pores and blackheads	Follow the 28-day program: reduce fat and oil intake to reduce sebum production; take a zinc supplement and possibly vitamin A; use skin-care products containing retinol and AHAs (it can take a long time for enlarged pores and blackheads to heal naturally)	A beautician, dermatologist, or cosmetic physician can advise on other options
Fungal infection on feet or nails; tinea	Use tea tree oil topically	See your medical doctor, a pharmacist, or a naturopathic doctor for stronger treatments
Melasma (chloasma, hyperpigmentation)	Skin-care products containing retinol and AHAs may marginally help; wear sunscreen with SPF 50 on affected areas (may resolve on its own if caused by pregnancy; home treatments may not be strong enough to remove all melasma)	A cosmetic physician or dermatologist can advise on other options

Skin problem	Treatments	Referrals
Menopause-related skin problems (dry and dull skin, reduced skin tone, poor skin immunity, wrinkles)	Follow the 28-day program: take a chromium supplement; take 1200 mg calcium daily, plus magnesium, copper, and vitamin D; use an active skin-care product plus a hydrating moisturizer applied on top	See your medical doctor for frequent checkups to rule out other causes
Pallor (pale, unhealthy-looking complexion)	Improve blood flow to the skin with daily exercise; check for biotin deficiency; refer to the Nutrient Deficiency Questionnaire (page 108); increase intake of alkalizing foods to improve blood flow (refer to Acid–Alkaline Food Charts, page 76)	See your doctor to rule out other factors
Pigmentation, hyperpigmentation, and mottled pigmentation	Use fade/bleach creams containing AHAs; wear SPF 50 sunscreen on affected areas (home treatments may not be strong enough to remove all pigmentation, especially after pregnancy)	A cosmetic physician or dermatologist can advise on other options
Psoriasis	Follow a fresh, healthy diet; avoid junk food; avoid cigarette smoke; learn to manage stress; avoid alcohol	Use water, sunlight, and oil therapy and liver cleansing (refer to the psoriasis chapter in The Healthy Skin Diet)
Rosacea	Daily exercise is essential	Limit histamine foods in the diet (refer to the rosacea chapter in The Healthy Skin Diet)
Rough skin	Exfoliate; take an omega-3 fish oil supplement or flaxseed oil daily; drink 8 glasses of filtered water daily; use skin-care products containing AHAs	A beautician or dermatologist can advise on other options
Sagging skin (age related, post-pregnancy, or from weight loss)	Follow the 28-day program: increase protein in the diet if necessary; exercise and use weights daily (see a personal trainer for a program to suit your needs); check for nutritional deficiencies, especially copper and zinc; take 1000 to 1200 mg of calcium daily	A cosmetic physician can advise on other options
Sensitive, dry skin	Follow the 28-day program: take an omega-3 fish oil supplement; avoid sulfites in skin care; use gentle skin-care products	
Slow wound healing	Follow the 28-day program: check for nutrient deficiencies	See your medical doctor

Skin problem	Treatments	Referrals
Spider veins and varicose veins	There is no natural way to reverse them, but you can limit further damage and reduce pain by avoiding standing up on hard surfaces for extended periods and by reducing saturated fat intake — avoid eating red meat, pork, and chicken skin	A cosmetic physician or vein specialist can effectively treat vein problems
Stretch marks	These can occur if you are zinc-deficient during pregnancy or during weight gain; it's hard to reverse, but products containing retinol and AHAs may help; to avoid future problems, take a zinc supplement or eat zinc-rich foods and vitamin C–rich foods; moisturize your skin daily	A cosmetic physician or dermatologist can advise on other options
Uneven skin tone	Follow the 28-day program: check for nutritional deficiencies; exercise daily; use skin-care products containing retinol and AHAs; correct with makeup	A cosmetic physician, beautician, or dermatologist can advise on other options
Wrinkles	Follow the 28-day program to reduce appearance of fine lines: check for nutritional deficiencies; take a calcium and omega-3 supplement or add flax seeds to your diet; avoid future sun damage by wearing a hat and sunscreen (SPF 50) daily to protect face, neck, hands, and feet (even on cloudy days)	A cosmetic physician or dermatologist can advise on other options
Yellow skin and eyes	Follow the 28-day program: reduce AGEs in your diet; check for nutritional deficiencies — refer to the Nutrient Deficiency Questionnaire (page 108); consuming large amounts of carrots can cause skin discoloration	See your doctor for a checkup to rule out other factors, such as liver problems

Part 1
Nurturing Younger Skin

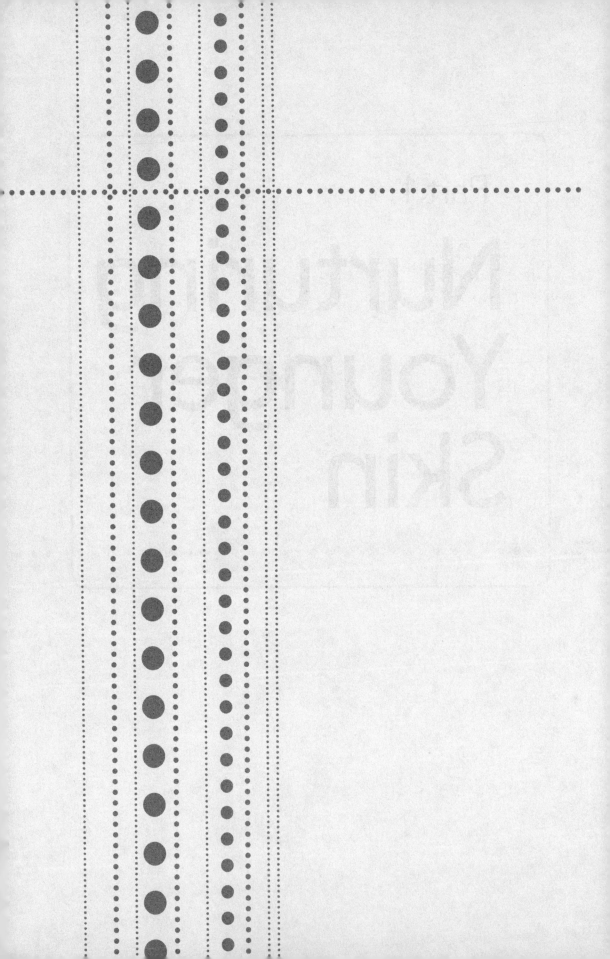

Chapter 1
Skin Basics

· ·

"Wrinkled was not one of the things I wanted to be when I grew up."

Beautiful skin is a blessing that you take for granted when you are young. Your skin is your largest organ (and the most visible one), and you walk around clothed in it every day of your life. Then you grow up and you begin to age. Your skin becomes drier and bumpier as wrinkles appear. This aging process does not need to happen. Now is the time to step up your health and skin-care routine, because healthy, younger-looking skin is more than just a pretty facade. It is central to your health.

Functions of the Skin

Your skin performs a wide range of important body functions that help keep you alive.
- Your skin is part of your immune system, acting as a barrier between the outside world and your organs, filtering out invading microbes and fungus, and expelling dangerous diseases, bacteria, and viruses.
- Your skin helps to regulate your body temperature so you don't overheat your internal organs.
- Your skin plays a major role in maintaining bone health.
- Your skin can show early signs of nutritional deficiencies, indicating that a change in diet is due.

Did You Know?
· · · · · · · · · · · · · · · · ·
Shedding Your Skin
- Every 40 minutes you shed about 1 million dead skin cells, and over a lifetime you'll shed enough skin to fill a suitcase.
- Between the ages of 30 and 80, the skin's cell turnover rate decreases by 30% to 50% (but you can increase this with the right skin-care routine).

Healthy, younger-looking skin is more than just a pretty facade. It is central to your health.

Anatomy of the Skin

The skin has three interacting layers: epidermis, dermis, and subcutaneous layers.

Epidermis

The epidermis is the outer (or dead) layer of your skin. It is thinnest on your eyelids, at $\frac{1}{1000}$ of an inch (0.05 mm), and thickest on your palms and soles, at approximately $\frac{3}{50}$ of an inch (1.5 mm). The epidermis itself contains five layers, which are mostly made up of cells that produce keratin, a tough and fibrous protein that forms a protective

Human Skin Components

New skin cells form at the bottom of the epidermis, and when they are ready, they move toward the stratum corneum. In normal, healthy skin, this trip takes about 4 weeks.

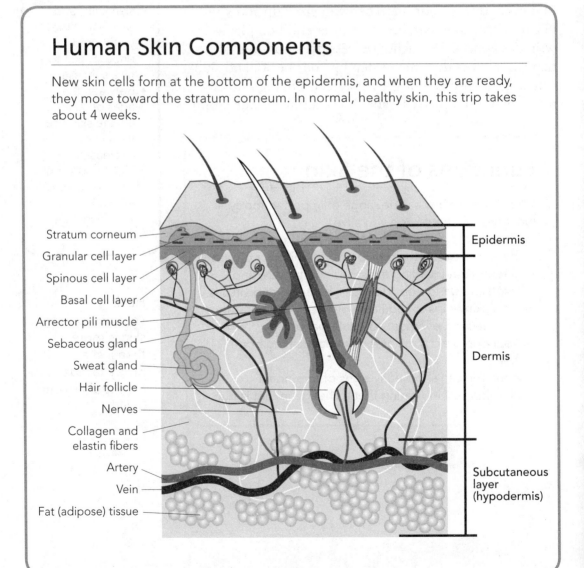

Stratum corneum
Granular cell layer
Spinous cell layer
Basal cell layer
Arrector pili muscle
Sebaceous gland
Sweat gland
Hair follicle
Nerves
Collagen and elastin fibers
Artery
Vein
Fat (adipose) tissue

Epidermis

Dermis

Subcutaneous layer (hypodermis)

layer. The column-shaped cells in the bottom layer push cells into higher layers — this skin-renewing trip takes about 28 days. The top layer of the epidermis, the stratum corneum (or skin barrier), is made of flat, dead cells that shed about every 2 weeks.

When the epidermis is functioning properly, the following youth-preserving properties are at optimal levels.

Properties	Functions	Source
Acid mantle: Your skin should have an acidic pH of approximately 5.5	Protects the skin from harmful microbes and candida overgrowth	Dietary skin lipids, unsaturated fatty acids, and amino acids from protein foods; use pH-balanced skin-care products
Sebum: Made up of oils and fatty acids secreted from sebaceous (oil) glands	Waterproof sealant: moisturizes the skin (overactive = acne; underactive = dry skin)	Beta-cryptoxanthin, a carotenoid in papaya, red bell pepper, paprika, pumpkin, and squash, increases sebum and skin hydration; zinc and vitamin A normalize overproduction
Sweat: Produced via sweat glands in the dermis	Flushes microbes from the surface of your skin; contains lysozyme, an enzyme that fights bacteria; assists with the removal of waste products from your body	As you age, sweat declines; daily exercise, enough to sweat, gives your skin a natural, healthy glow
Skin pigment: Formed in the epidermis by melanin and hemoglobin (blood)	Helps to protect your skin from ultraviolet (UV) rays and reduce the risk of skin cancer	As you age, liver spots and uneven pigmentation can occur

Loss of Elasticity

Interlocking fingerlike waves join the epidermis to the dermis, which is the deeper layer of skin. This important junction allows nutrients and oxygen to travel from the inner layers to the outer layer of the skin so it stays healthy. When levels of hormones, such as estrogen, decline, the fingerlike junctions flatten and nutrient exchange slows, causing a loss of elasticity in the skin. However, no matter what your hormones are doing (or not doing), daily exercise can help to manually improve blood flow to the surface of your skin.

Dermis

The deeper layer of skin is the dermis. It's like the soil in a garden, situated below the surface, with the all-important jobs of maintaining the skin's structure and supplying nutrients and fluids. The dermis is a thick layer containing bundles of collagen fibers and coarse elastic fibers made of elastin, which enable the skin to stretch and return to its original shape. The dermis also contains sweat glands, hair follicles, veins, and hyaluronic acid, which attracts and holds water. Wrinkles appear when changes occur to the deeper layers of the dermis.

When the dermis is functioning properly, the following four youth-preserving properties are at optimal levels.

Collagen

Collagen is like the glue that keeps your skin together. It's an amazing protein structure in the skin that twines in a triple ropelike formation, called a helix, so it is extra strong and durable — on a weight-per-weight basis, collagen is nearly as strong as steel. More than one-third of collagen is made up of the amino acid glycine, another third is proline, and a small proportion consists of lysine and other amino acids. These amino acids are found in protein-containing foods, such as fish, eggs, meats, beans, nuts, and seeds. For healthy collagen production in the skin, your diet needs to be rich in protein, vitamin C, iron, zinc, and manganese. As you age, your body produces fewer collagen fibers, especially in the upper dermis.

Elastin

If you were to pick up an elastic band and stretch it around a jar and then later take it off, the elastic band would snap back to its original shape and size. The elastic fibers within your dermis should also stretch (up to 150% of their relaxed length without breaking) and return to their original shape.

Hyaluronic Acid

In normal skin, glycosaminoglycans (GAGs), such as hyaluronic acid, are found between collagen and elastic fibers in the dermal layer. Hyaluronic acid is also found in the epidermis of younger skin but disappears as you age.

Did You Know?

Like Lycra

Elastin is a protein found within coarse elastic fibers in the dermal layer of the skin, which branch together to give the skin strength and flexibility. Like a Lycra swimsuit that loses tautness over time, your skin can lose some of its elasticity during the aging process.

It is hydrophilic, which means it attracts water, protecting collagen and elastin from becoming rigid.

Smoking cigarettes decreases the amount of hyaluronic acid in your body. You can increase hyaluronic acid naturally by adding its main building block, glucosamine, to your diet. Magnesium and zinc are also needed to manufacture hyaluronic acid. Some researchers believe that traditional societies who age well do so because their traditional diet, rich in root vegetables, supplies plenty of magnesium and zinc for the production of hyaluronic acid.

Blood Supply Rich with Nutrients

A healthy blood supply to the skin gives your complexion an attractive, healthy glow. The bloodstream carries oxygen and nutrients to the skin for the maintenance, repair, and building of new skin cells. As you age, the walls of blood vessels in the dermis become thicker and more rigid, and if your diet (or your digestion) is poor, your skin may not receive enough nutrients. The first indicator is a dull complexion, and over time, problems — such as skin abnormalities, premature aging, and poor wound healing (and skin ulcers, in the case of diabetes) — can occur.

> A healthy blood supply to the skin gives your complexion an attractive, healthy glow.

Subcutaneous

Beneath the dermis lies the subcutaneous layer, which contains fat cells. Your fat cells provide cushioning and insulation to protect the body, and they plump the skin so it looks younger. As you age, these fat cells get smaller in areas such as the face. If you are thin, your face can age faster because you have fewer fat stores to pad your skin and minimize the appearance of wrinkles.

In areas such as the thighs, buttocks, and stomach, the opposite can occur. The subcutaneous layer thickens (predominantly in women) so that fat cells protrude into the dermis and cause cellulite.

Did You Know?

Plump cells
Your fat cells provide cushioning and insulation to protect the body, and they plump the skin so it looks younger.

Cellulite

Cellulite is considered a cosmetic defect, not a disease or disorder. It appears as lumpy skin and is caused by disordered fat cells in the subcutaneous layer.

Largely thanks to genetics, women have a tougher battle with cellulite. However, female athletes usually have no

FAQ

Q. Why do women get cellulite more often than men?

A. Around 5% of men develop cellulite and up to 90% of older women will have it at some point in their lives. Women are more likely than men to develop cellulite because they have three main structural differences in the skin:

1. The epidermis, or outer layer, of the skin is thinner in women (men naturally have tougher skin, and women have lovely, soft skin).
2. The dermis layer of the skin is a lot thinner in women, and this progressively worsens with aging, eventually allowing fat cells to protrude into this layer.
3. Women have more fat cells and subcutaneous tissue (increased cushioning to help women survive childbirth).

The Skin Pinch Test

During a pinch test, fat cells can protrude into the dermis in the buttocks and thigh region, and occasionally in the stomach area.

Exercising frequently is one of the keys to minimizing or preventing cellulite; another is taking a calcium citrate supplement. Research also shows that massage helps reduce water retention, improve lymphatic drainage, and increase collagen synthesis in sufferers of cellulite.

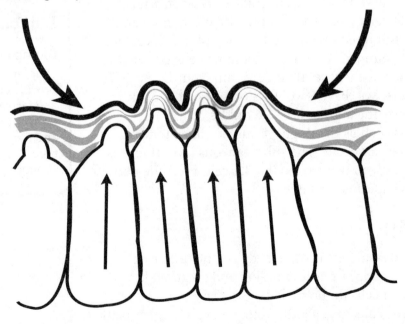

FAQ

Q. I am going through menopause. What can I do to reduce the symptoms of aging?

A. Menopause is a perfectly normal milestone in a woman's life, when menstruation ceases and you are no longer fertile. It begins with perimenopause, where estrogen levels gradually drop. Low estrogen levels can promote inflammation and decrease collagen production in the skin, and skin elasticity decreases by 0.55% per year after perimenopause. Calcium supplementation is essential during menopause because low estrogen causes calcium deficiency, which contributes to loss of skin elasticity. Epidermal ridges also flatten, which increases skin fragility and hampers nutrient distribution in the skin — this can cause your complexion to look dull. However, this is greatly improved with daily exercise, which flushes the skin with nutrient-rich blood (provided you also eat a healthy, nutrient-rich diet). For information on treating menopause-related skin problems, refer to the Quick Guide to Skin Problems on page 12.

cellulite, even as they age, and it's from these women that we can gain hope and also a bit of insight into how to avoid or reduce cellulite. Research shows that weight loss (if it's required) causes fat cells to retract out of the dermis.

Skin Messengers

Your endocrine system, comprising your hormones and glands, is heavily involved in the aging process. The endocrine system produces and regulates hormones, which can drastically decline as you age. Hormones are used to regulate growth, mood, metabolism, sexual and reproductive function, and collagen production in the skin, to name a few.

> Hormones are used to regulate growth, mood, metabolism, sexual and reproductive function, and collagen production in the skin, to name a few.

Estrogens are the main sex hormone in women, but they are present in small amounts in men, too. Estrogens increase glycosaminoglycans (GAGs), such as hyaluronic acid, which softens and hydrates the skin and helps to maintain structural quality (which is why women have softer skin than men). Estrogens have anti-inflammatory properties and they play a role in the network of collagen and elastin in your skin, helping to increase collagen production and promote healthy hair.

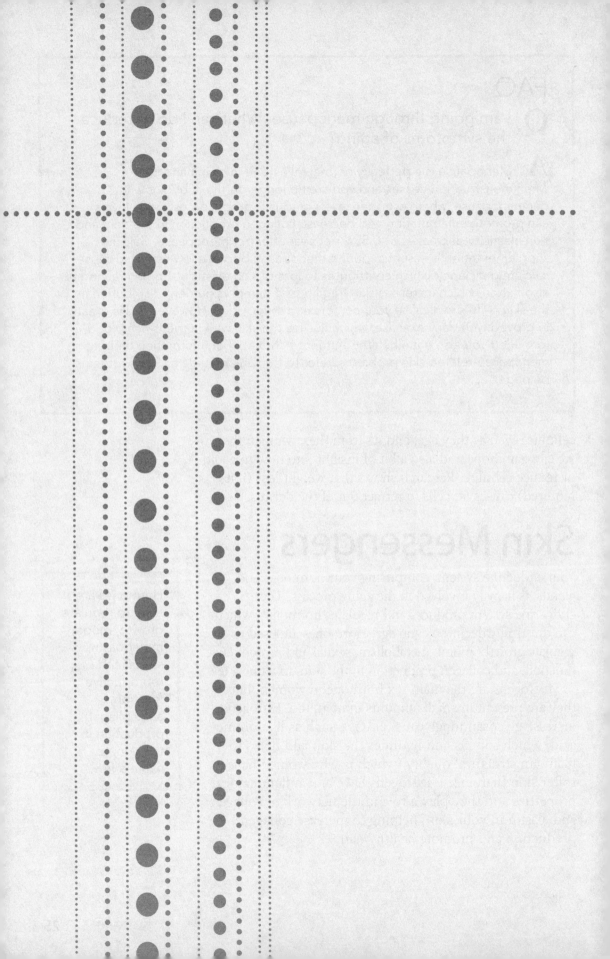

Chapter 2
AGEs and Antioxidants

● ●

Skin ages because of intrinsic and extrinsic factors. Your genes are thought to influence intrinsic aging, such as your hormone levels naturally declining as you age. Skin that ages intrinsically, with little or no extrinsic assaults, is generally fairly smooth with some noticeable expression lines, pigment changes, graying hairs, and skin dryness.

Extrinsic aging is largely influenced by external factors. These are the habits you can often limit or avoid, such as frequent sun exposure, poor diet, and cigarette smoking. Extrinsic aging contributes to deep wrinkles, frown lines, dehydrated skin, rosacea, and sallow skin. Aging may not be totally avoidable, but you can certainly avoid or limit factors that cause extrinsic aging.

AGEs

Advanced glycation end products, or AGEs, appear to be a major factor in skin aging and have been implicated in various diseases, such as diabetes and heart disease. AGEs are the product of sugar metabolism, exposure to ultraviolet (UV) light, and cooking practices. Glucose and other sugars are involved as they attach, or cross-link, to proteins in collagen and form the advanced glycation end products. This cross-linking stiffens collagen and elastin fibers and renders them incapable of easy repair. AGEs can also accumulate in the body through UV radiation from the sun, and they can be consumed in your diet (they are plentiful in fried meats and some other foods). High consumption of dietary AGEs contributes to tissue damage and impaired wound healing of the skin.

> **Did You Know?**
> ....
> **AGEs Contribute to Aging Skin**
> Advanced glycation end products (AGEs), the product of sugar metabolism, exposure to ultraviolet light, and high-heat cooking practices, appear to be a major factor in skin aging, contributing to tissue damage and impaired wound healing.

Glycation Process

Think of AGEs as brownish spots — like sticky toffee — that grab onto collagen when there is lots of sugar in your blood. Not all AGE-rich foods are brown, but when you eat browned foods (from frying and roasting), you are consuming a higher dose of AGEs. When your skin goes brown from exposure to the sun, AGEs are forming, too. Keep in mind that your skin doesn't necessarily need to go brown to be accumulating AGEs — fair-skinned people are at an increased risk due to low pigment, and dark-skinned people may have added protection against sun-induced AGEs.

Glycation — the chemical process that generates AGEs — increases in frequency as you age. There are three main ways AGEs can form within your body: the oxidation of glucose caused by free radicals; the peroxidation of fats, which are also damaged by free radicals (see Free Radical Skin Aging, page 30); and via the Maillard reaction.

Maillard Reaction

The formation of AGEs via the Maillard reaction happens in three stages:

1. This is a slow process that relies on sugars being present in the blood, and the first step takes place within hours of ingesting sugars, such as glucose. If the concentration of glucose subsequently declines, this initial reaction is reversible.

2. If glucose stays elevated, the second stage occurs. Over a period of days, early glycation products form. This phase is reversible if your blood sugar levels decline (meaning that you give your body a break from consuming sugars and processed carbohydrates, the culprits that lead to high glucose).

3. If the early glycation products accumulate, over a period of weeks, they form cross-link proteins, which are not reversible. The brownish end products are called AGEs, and they literally age you.

Associated Conditions of AGEs

- Aging
- Alzheimer's disease
- Atherosclerosis
- Cataracts and other eye problems
- Diabetes
- Elevated blood sugar levels
- End-stage renal disease
- Inflammatory skin changes
- Loss of bone density
- Loss of muscle mass
- Parkinson's disease
- Reduced muscle function and strength
- Reduced skin elasticity
- Rheumatoid arthritis
- Yellowing of the skin

Cross-Linking of Collagen and AGE Accumulation in the Skin

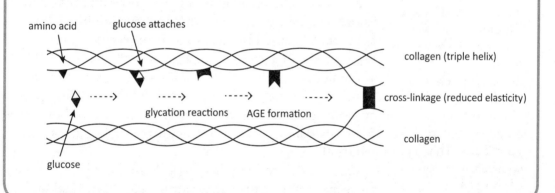

Cross-Linking

AGEs accumulate in the dermal layer of your skin partially by attaching themselves to collagen proteins. A collagen fiber normally forms a springlike coil structure and maintains skin elasticity in combination with elastin fibers. However, when AGEs attach to collagen, the cross-links lock the collagen fibers in place and skin elasticity is reduced.

The Research...

- The accumulation of AGEs in the dermis layer of the skin changes the optical characteristics of cells, causing reduced skin transparency and skin yellowing.

- AGEs cause damage because of their pro-oxidant and inflammatory actions, and the skin can appear red and blotchy.

- AGEs and the cross-linking of collagen cause the stiffening of blood vessels and the loss of muscle mass and strength as you age.

Free Radical Skin Aging

Free radicals are best described as unstable molecules or "one-armed thieves" — they have a missing "arm" (an electron) and they seek to fill this missing space by stealing an electron from a nearby cell in your body. This causes oxidation of the cell, resulting in DNA damage or cell death.

A slice of cut apple soon begins to brown, raw meat past its use-by date turns brown, and rust appears in an old car due to a process called oxidation. In fact, corrosion, rust, and oxidation all mean the same thing. Oxidation in the human body can be caused by AGEs and by molecules called free radicals. Free radicals are best described as unstable molecules or "one-armed thieves" — they have a missing "arm" (an electron) and they seek to fill this missing space by stealing an electron from a nearby cell in your body. This causes oxidation of the cell, resulting in DNA damage or cell death.

Your body produces free radicals all the time, when you move and eat, and they are a normal part of the making and functioning of your cells. In this way, they are partly unavoidable. However, excess free radicals can become a problem and lead to rapid aging of the skin.

Free radicals set off a chain of events in the body that degrades collagen and elastic fibers. They also trigger the overproduction of melanin, leading to mottled skin pigmentation and other common signs of aging.

Antioxidant Heroes

Although free radicals cannot be totally avoided, free radical damage in the skin can be greatly reduced by a diet and skin-care regimen rich in antioxidants. Antioxidants include vitamins A, C, and E, alpha-lipoic acid, anthocyanins, beta-carotene, lycopene, zinc, selenium, coenzyme Q10, and resveratrol, to name a few.

Antioxidants protect your skin cells by donating one of their electrons to a free radical — so the free radical can no longer damage a nearby skin cell. By stopping the chain reaction of destruction caused by free radicals, antioxidants become oxidized themselves. It's better them than you!

Antioxidants are supplied by a healthy diet rich in vegetables and exotic grains and fruit, and antioxidant-rich skin-care products also have a protective effect on the skin.

There are a range of antioxidant nutrients, such as vitamin C and resveratrol, that can break down some types of AGEs in the body. However, the bad news is that there is no agent that can break down the most common AGE, glucosepane, which is made when glucose attaches to collagen. Glucosepane levels are 10 to 1,000 times higher in human tissue than any other cross-linking AGE, and the only way to decrease levels of this harmful molecule is to reduce sugars in the diet.

> Free radical damage in the skin can be greatly reduced by a diet and skin-care regimen rich in antioxidants.

AGE Food List

The following table lists foods from lowest to highest amount of dietary AGEs contained. If you consume 3½ ounces (100 g) of anything in the "very high" column on the right-hand side, you could exceed the recommended daily intake (which should not exceed 5000 to 8000 kilounits, or kU). Favor foods in the first two columns — "low" and "low-medium." Avoid everything listed in the "high" and "very high" columns.

The table is based on AGE kU per 3½ ounce (100 g), N-(Carboxymethyl)lysine (CLM) content only — other types of AGEs might be present.

Low-AGE foods: 0–99	Low- to medium-AGE foods: 100–999	High-AGE foods: 1000–4999	Very-high-AGE foods: 5000+
Most fruits	Almonds, raw	Almonds, blanched or roasted	Most cheeses
Most vegetables	Avocado	Chicken, ground, fried	Bacon
Bran flakes	Bagel	Cookies	Beef kebab
Chicken soup	Chicken, marinated with lemon	Cottage cheese	Beef, ground, fried
Egg, poached	Chicken, poached with lemon	Crabmeat, fried	Butter
Egg, scrambled over low heat for 2 minutes	Chicken, steamed with lemon	Egg, fried	Canola oil
Egg white	Coconut milk	Figs, dried	Chicken kebab
Ketchup	Corned beef	Granola bars	Chicken nuggets
Lentil soup	Egg, scrambled over high heat for 1 minute	Lamb, marinated	Chicken, deep-fried
Oatmeal	Eggplant, grilled or broiled	Mozzarella, reduced-fat	Chicken, roasted
Omelet, cooked over low heat	Fish, steamed in foil with lemon	Salmon, fried	Cottonseed oil
Porridge	Granola	Shrimp, fried	Cream cheese
Potatoes	Hummus	Tofu, fried, grilled or broiled	Deli meats
Rice	Kidney beans	Veal, stewed	Grilled cheese sandwich
Rolled oats	Pasta		Hamburger (beef)
Soy sauce	Pistachios		Hot dogs
Tamari	Pitas		Margarine
Tea, black or herbal	Plums		Mayonnaise
Vegetable juice	Raisins		Peanut butter
Vegetable soup	Salad dressing		Peanuts
Veggie burger	Salmon, canned, raw or smoked		Pizza (store-bought)
Whole-grain bread, untoasted	Soy burger		Roast beef
	Tofu, raw		Sausages
	Trout, raw		Sesame oil
	Vegetables, grilled or broiled		Steak, fried

The Research...

- The antioxidant carnosine protects against glycation because it blocks the cross-linking of sugars with collagen.

- Lab studies showed that alpha-lipoic acid reversed collagen glycation due to its antioxidant action and its reducing effect on blood sugar levels.

- A study found that cinnamon, ginger, cloves, marjoram, rosemary, and tarragon all have a protective effect against AGEs because they contain protective phenolic antioxidants.

- Antioxidant flavonoids, such as luteolin, quercetin, and rutin, from onions and other vegetables inhibit various stages of AGE formation.

For younger skin, avoid AGEs and eat antioxidant-rich foods.

Swap This for That

Pioneering AGE researchers Dr. Jaime Uribarri and Dr. Helen Vlassara recommend that your daily AGE consumption should not exceed 5000 to 8000 kilounits. However, the typical Western diet is very rich in AGEs and the average AGE consumption is approximately 15,000 and up to 25,000 daily (those who consumed more than 10,000 were found by the researchers to be prone to being overweight or had diabetes and other health problems).

The following tables list some typical food choices for meals throughout the day, along with AGE amounts. These are then followed by low-AGE alternatives.

Total daily AGEs for #1 meals = 24,554
Total daily AGEs for #2 meals = 3064

Breakfast #1: High-AGE

Food	AGE content (in kU)
2 eggs (3½ oz/100 g), fried	2749
2 slices white bread (2 oz/60 g), toasted, with 2 tsp (10 mL) butter	2712
1 cup (250 mL) coffee (from pot of brewed coffee that has been on a heating plate for 1 hour)	34
TOTAL:	5495

Breakfast #2: Low-AGE

Food	AGE content (in kU)
2 eggs, poached* (3½ oz/100 g)	90
2 slices whole wheat bread (3½ oz/100 g), toasted, no butter or margarine	120
Bowl of porridge	18
1 cup (250 mL) tea	5
TOTAL:	233

* 2 eggs scrambled on low heat with minimal olive oil is also a good option, with 97 kU per 3½ oz/100 g.

Lunch #1: High-AGE

Food	AGE content (in kU)
Chicken (3½ oz/100 g), grilled	5200
2 slices white bread (2 oz/60 g), with 2 tsp (10 mL) butter	2417
1 cup (250 mL) coffee (from pot of brewed coffee that has been on a heating plate for 1 hour)	34
TOTAL:	7651

Lunch #2: Low-AGE

Food	AGE content (in kU)
Chicken (3½ oz/100 g), poached with lemon	861
2 slices whole wheat bread (3½ oz/100 g), no butter or margarine	53
2 tsp (10 mL) avocado, used as a spread	158
1 cup (250 mL) mixed salad leaves	17
1 cup (250 mL) coffee, freshly brewed	6
1 apple	15
TOTAL:	1110

Dinner #1: High-AGE

Food	AGE content (in kU)
Steak (3½ oz/100 g), fried in oil	10,058
French fries (3½ oz/100 g), homemade	694
1 cup (250 mL) hot chocolate for dessert	656
TOTAL:	11,408

Dinner #2: Low-AGE

Food	AGE content (in kU)
Salmon (3½ oz/100 g), poached or steamed*	1477
Vegetables (3½ oz/100 g), grilled	226
Rice (3½ oz/100 g)	9
Banana (3½ oz/100 g) for dessert	9
TOTAL:	1721

* No data showing AGE content if pre-marinated

AGE Questionnaire

Fill out the following questionnaire to see if you're exposed to increased levels of AGEs. Circle the most correct answer (YES / SOMETIMES / NO) for each question. Your score for each answer is in parentheses. For example, in Question 2, if you eat puffed/flaked breakfast cereal three times weekly, your answer is YES and your score is 10. Write your score in the space provided to the right.

YES = weekly or daily
SOMETIMES = monthly or occasionally
NO = never or very rarely

Part A	Score
1. How old are you? Under 20 (0) 45 to 54 (40) 20 to 34 (10) 55 to 64 (50) 35 to 44 (30) 65 or above (60)	
2. Do you eat commercial breakfast cereal? (These are the cereals that are crunchy, crispy, toasted, flaked, or puffed, not including raw oats or porridge.) YES (10) SOMETIMES (5) NO (0)	
3. Do you eat toasted bread with butter or margarine? YES (15) SOMETIMES (10) NO (0)	
4. Do you eat toasted bread with no butter or margarine? YES (5) SOMETIMES (2) NO (0)	
5. Do you like to overcook your toast so it is burnt on the edges? YES (10) SOMETIMES (5) NO (0)	
6. Do you eat fish and/or other seafood? YES (10) SOMETIMES (5) NO (0)	
7. Do you eat chicken that is fried, baked, stir-fried, roasted, or grilled? (If you only eat chicken that is poached or boiled, give yourself 10 points.) YES (15) SOMETIMES (10) NO (0)	
8. Do you eat red meat, such as beef, steak, and lamb? YES (18) SOMETIMES (12) NO (0)	
9. Do you eat pork, such as pork chops, bacon, ham, and roast pork with crackling? YES (18) SOMETIMES (12) NO (0)	
10. Do you eat fried foods, such as fish and chips, chicken nuggets, fish sticks, spring rolls, and french fries? YES (24) SOMETIMES (15) NO (0)	

Part A (continued)	Score
11. Do you roast, grill, fry, or barbecue animal protein foods (such as red meat, eggs, seafood, and poultry) using butter, margarine, or vegetable oil (such as canola, olive, sunflower, or coconut)? YES (20) SOMETIMES (12) NO (0)	
12. Do you consume dairy products, such as milk, cheese, yogurt, butter, and ice cream? YES (15) SOMETIMES (10) NO (0)	
13. Do you eat pastries, toasted muesli bars, doughnuts, or other toasted or browned bakery items? YES (15) SOMETIMES (10) NO (0)	
14. Do you eat bacon, sausages, or hot dogs? YES (22) SOMETIMES (15) NO (0)	
15. Do you eat deli meats, such as ham, turkey, salami, or Spam? YES (22) SOMETIMES (15) NO (0)	
16. Do you eat pizza or fast-food hamburgers? YES (24) SOMETIMES (15) NO (0)	
17. Do you add sweeteners (such as artificial sweetener, sugar, or honey) to foods, beverages (such as coffee or tea), cereals, or desserts? (The "NO" value is 5 points to account for the natural fruit sugars and glucose from some vegetables.) YES (20) SOMETIMES (10) NO (5)	
18. Do you overeat or are you considered overweight? YES (20) SOMETIMES (10) NO (0)	
19. Do you have diabetes or any of the following: high blood sugar, Alzheimer's disease, cardiovascular disease, Parkinson's disease, end-stage renal disease, rheumatoid arthritis, or cataracts or other degenerative eye diseases? YES (28) NO (0)	
20. Do you drink more than 3 servings of alcohol weekly? YES (20) SOMETIMES (15) NO (0)	
21. Do you smoke cigarettes? YES (22) SOMETIMES (18) NO (0)	
22. Do you tan your skin through sun exposure or sun beds, or do you spend prolonged time in the sun without sunscreen? (The "NO" value is worth 10 points to allow for incidental sun exposure.) YES (30) SOMETIMES (20) NO (10)	
Add up your total score for Part A TOTAL:	

Part B	Score
1. How often do you exercise? Daily (10) 1 to 2 days/week (2) 3 to 6 days/week (5) Rarely or never (0)	
2. How often do you eat purple fruits and vegetables (such as eggplant, blueberries, red cabbage, red onion, purple carrots, and purple mixed lettuce)? Daily (10) 1 to 2 days/week (2) 3 to 6 days/week (5) Rarely or never (0)	
3. How often do you eat salads or steamed vegetables (a serving size of at least 1 cup/250 mL)? Daily (10) 1 to 2 days/week (2) 3 to 6 days/week (5) Rarely or never (0)	
4. How often do you eat raw oats or porridge with fruit? Daily (5) 1 to 2 days/week (1) 3 to 6 days/week (3) Rarely or never (0)	
5. How often do you use fresh lemon and lime in drinks, cooking, meat marinades, etc.? Daily (10) 1 to 2 days/week (3) 3 to 6 days/week (5) Rarely or never (0)	
6. How often do you drink antioxidant-rich teas, such as ginger, chai (leaf tea, not powdered chai latte), green tea, or peppermint or other herbal teas? Daily (5) 1 to 2 days/week (1) 3 to 6 days/week (3) Rarely or never (0)	
7. How often do you add cinnamon, cloves, or curry powder to your meals? Daily (10) 1 to 2 days/week (3) 3 to 6 days/week (5) Rarely or never (0)	
8. Do you have naturally dark skin that is resistant to wrinkles and sun damage? No (0) Olive skin, Italian, etc. (10) Darker skin, African-American, African, Indian, etc. (20)	
Add up your total score for Part B TOTAL:	
Calculation Now subtract your Part B score from your Part A score. For example, if your Part A score was 120 and your Part B score was 75, then your final score would be 45. Your aim on this program is to score as close to 0 as possible. This book will show you how to achieve this. Keep in mind that AGEs also accumulate as you age, so the older you are, the more careful you have to be with your diet and lifestyle.	FINAL TOTAL

Recap

- Advanced glycation end products (AGEs) are obtained in three ways: they are formed inside the body (due to the natural aging process and/or the presence of sugars), they accumulate from sun exposure, and they are supplied by your diet.

- Low-AGE diets reduce inflammation and oxidative damage.

- Meats, cheeses, fast food, and fats contain the highest dietary AGEs.

- Vegetables, fruits, beans, and whole grains are low in dietary AGEs.

- High cooking temperatures and longer cooking times increase AGEs in foods.

- Cooking with liquids and at lower temperatures greatly reduce the formation of AGEs.

- Processed and takeout foods contain more AGEs than raw or homemade foods.

- Free radicals can lead to rapid aging of the skin. Antioxidants can counteract free radicals.

Chapter 3
The
Dirty Dozen

● ●

When it comes to sabotaging the health of your skin, there is a range of factors that can fast-track wrinkling, mottled pigmentation, and other signs of aging. The Dirty Dozen — aptly named because AGEs are brownish in color — includes foods that elevate AGE formation and foods that promote glycation, the chemical process that creates AGEs. The Dirty Dozen also includes foods that are rich sources of dietary AGEs, which attack collagen and contribute to organ, blood vessel, and tissue damage.

The buildup in the body of too many AGEs is linked to diabetes, heart disease, and problems with kidney function. Studies also suggest AGEs can harm the immune system and promote arthritis. You may not be able to prevent the biological aging process (which involves some AGE formation and hormonal changes, and so on), but research shows you can simply eat fewer AGEs to improve your health, skin, and longevity. Here are the top factors, the Dirty Dozen, that increase AGEs in the body.

> The buildup in the body of too many AGEs is linked to diabetes, heart disease, and problems with kidney function.

FAQ

Q. Are fruit sugars bad for me?

A. Fruit contains fruit sugars, chiefly fructose, which can be used by the body to form AGEs. However, avoiding fruit is not the answer to long-term health — quite the opposite. Most fruits are rich in important antioxidants, which protect against AGEs and free radical damage. A diet devoid of fruit causes the antioxidant levels in your skin to plummet, and this puts you at an increased risk of diseases, such as skin cancer and scurvy, plus it can leave you more vulnerable to sunburn and premature aging. It is important to consume 2 to 3 servings of fruit daily for good health.

1. Sugar

Although some health experts say sugar is an empty-calorie food that is harmless in moderation, it appears they may be mistaken. If you want younger-looking skin, new research suggests you skip the sugar and choose healthier options. Sugar consumption contributes to a loss of skin elasticity and can trigger the appearance of acne and premature wrinkles. A diet high in sugar may also shorten your lifespan. Scientists from the University of California in San Francisco reported that excess sugar consumption is indirectly responsible for 35 million deaths annually worldwide because it significantly increases the risk of AGE-related diseases, such as diabetes and heart disease.

Sugars Commonly Found in Processed Food Products and Recipes

- Agave nectar
- Barley malt
- Beet sugar
- Cane sugar
- Caramel
- Corn sweetener
- Corn syrup
- Corn syrup solids (in baby formulas)
- Crystalline fructose
- D-mannose
- Dextran
- Dextrin
- Dextrose
- Ethyl maltol
- Florida Crystals
- Fructose
- Fruit juice
- Galactose
- Glucose
- Golden syrup
- High-fructose corn syrup (HFCS)
- Honey
- Lactose (milk sugar)
- Malt syrup
- Maltodextrin
- Maltose
- Mannitol
- Maple syrup
- Molasses
- Rice malt syrup
- Sorbitol
- Sucrose
- Treacle

The Research...

- Sugars, such as glucose, attach to collagen and elastic fibers and form advanced glycation end products. This cross-linking stiffens collagen and elastin fibers, making them difficult to repair.

- A low-sugar diet reduces the sugar level within the skin.

On average, Americans consume $27\frac{1}{2}$ teaspoons (136 mL) of hidden (and not-so-hidden) sugars every day, according to the U.S. Sugar Association. The annual sugar consumption in most Western countries is a staggering 110 lbs (50 kg) per person (that is 50 large bags of sugar).

FAQ

Q. I'm always craving sugar, bread, and alcohol. What should I do?

A. All three of these products supply the body with glucose for energy, but they are not in a desirable form that will give you a steady supply. You will soon crave more — an unhealthy cycle that is bad for your skin! Sugar cravings can indicate a number of concerns:

- Your body may be low in vitamin C, which is concentrated in sweet fruits (thus the biological craving for something sweet).
- If you have just eaten a salty meal, your body's electrolytes may be out of balance and your body is craving potassium — from fruit. The correct salt and potassium levels in your body are essential for the normal function of your cells and organs — so if you happen to eat a salty meal, grab a potassium-rich banana, peach, or papaya for dessert.
- You may have blood sugar issues, requiring chromium or cinnamon in the diet (which, to be most effective, must be consumed at the same time as eating carbohydrates).
- Lack of sleep, overworking, and skipping meals can cause sugar cravings.

Cravings for bread and other carbohydrates can indicate the need for a chromium and magnesium supplement, to help with blood sugar control. Cravings for alcohol can indicate the need for magnesium (and counseling, if necessary). If you have an insatiable craving for sugar or carbohydrates, eat quality low-glycemic-index grains, such as Omega Muesli (page 166), or grab a piece of antioxidant-rich fruit — 2 to 3 servings daily is recommended. Fruit is a guilt-free way to have a sweet treat and get your daily dose of AGE-reducing super-nutrients at the same time. The best fruits for younger skin are listed in the handy shopping guide on page 159.

Artificial Sweeteners

Artificial sweeteners include aspartame, saccharine, sucralose, and acesulfame potassium. Americans consume more than 24 lbs (10 kg) of artificial sweeteners per person each year. However, researchers have found that artificial sweeteners can lead to increased hunger and weight gain because they stimulate the release of the hormone insulin, which causes the accumulation of body fat. There are also concerns about the long-term safety of consuming large amounts of these artificial chemicals. Artificial sweeteners are not a healthy alternative to sugars and they are not a part of the 28-day program.

FAQ

Q. Carbohydrates are broken down into glucose. Should I avoid all carbs in order to avoid sugars?

A. Some glucose in the diet is essential for mental function and energy. Therefore, total carbohydrate avoidance is not recommended, and it can be harmful to your health in the long term. But there are some carbs your body could do without. Unhealthy carbohydrate foods that are overly processed and supply your body with too much glucose and too quickly are the ones to avoid — such as white flour, white bread, biscuits, cakes, and other foods high on the glycemic index (GI). These spike your blood sugar and increase AGE formation.

Other carbohydrate foods are essential to good health. Lower-GI carbohydrates — sweet potato, peas, rolled oats, and some other whole grains — give your body a steady and gradual supply of glucose, which is the "food" your brain uses for mental function. These are also your body's main source of energy. Without a slow and steady supply, you could experience energy crashes and sugar cravings, and you would feel foggy-brained and incredibly tired. Whole-grain carbohydrates, such as rolled oats, spelt, and quinoa, also give your body an important supply of fiber for bowel health — without enough dietary fiber, you would be frequently constipated and more likely to suffer skin breakouts. Some, such as red quinoa and sweet potato, are also a rich source of antioxidants and therefore fight AGE formation.

The Glycemic Index

The glycemic index, or GI, is a measure of how foods affect your blood glucose levels. You might know these as "blood sugar levels." Proteins and fats don't usually affect blood sugar; it is specifically a food's carbohydrate content that causes a spike in the sugars present in your blood (which is why you can feel a pleasant energy high when you eat sugar or high-GI foods, such as potato chips).

Low-GI foods fall in the range of 0 to 55, medium-GI foods fall between 56 and 69, and high-GI foods are above 70. For example, white bread has a GI of at least 70. Basmati rice is 58, which is a better choice than jasmine rice, which has a GI of 109. Low-GI foods are digested at a slower rate, so they release glucose into your bloodstream gradually. This is ideal, and will help you to feel fuller for longer and will give you a steady supply of energy in between meals. High-GI foods, such as puffed cereals (including puffed rice and amaranth), white bread (especially flatbread), and other white flour products, are digested rapidly and flood your bloodstream with large amounts of glucose.

In the short term, the high-GI foods give you a "high" feeling because glucose boosts energy, but — like all highs — it does not last, and you will soon crave that glucose buzz and feel hungrier than normal. Overeating can result. High-GI foods can also lead to energy slumps where you crave sugar as a quick fix. Over time, these glucose highs can damage blood vessels, stress the pancreas (the organ that dishes out insulin), cause weight gain, prematurely age the skin, and cause an increase of AGEs in the body. When eating carbs, favor lower-GI choices, such as basmati rice or sushi rice (instead of high-GI jasmine or white rice), and sourdough bread (instead of regular white bread). Add cinnamon to oats, quinoa, and curry dishes because cinnamon has a blood sugar–lowering effect (more on this later).

> High-GI foods give you a "high" feeling because glucose boosts energy, but — like all highs — it does not last, and you will soon crave that glucose buzz and feel hungrier than normal.

2. UV Exposure

The majority of sun damage happens during incidental activities. When waiting for your child at the school gate, driving your car, mowing the lawn, walking to the local shop, getting the mail — these kinds of activities account for two-thirds of your sunlight exposure. There is no better solution than to become a hat person and to wear a hat daily in order to protect your face.

Research shows that frequent UV exposure is the number one cause of wrinkles, but you don't need a study to confirm this. Just look at the skin on your buttocks (or an area that has not seen the sun) and compare it to your hands and you will see a remarkable difference in skin quality. Wrinkles are mostly found on sun-exposed skin — the face, chest, arms, knees, and hands.

Children attending primary school in Australia have a "No hat, no play" rule when outside, so they will probably grow up with younger skin than previous generations. However, it is never too late to start protecting your skin from the sun. By the time you are 18, your skin has only been exposed to less than 25% of your lifetime UV dose, which means that most of your UV-induced skin damage transpires during adulthood.

The Research...

- Sun exposure causes the formation of AGEs in the skin, and these paralyze collagen fibers and reduce skin elasticity.

- In normal skin, glycosaminoglycans (GAGs) are found between collagen and elastic fibers to offer support and hydration. After chronic sun exposure, GAGs move away from these fibers and hang in a different location, resulting in skin that is drier and prone to wrinkling.

- Exposing skin to the sun triggers the appearance of matrix metalloproteinases (MMPs), which degrade collagen and elastic fibers and play a role in skin aging. The good news is that a mixture of antioxidants, beta-carotene, and lycopene in the diet, consumed on a daily basis, can decrease harmful MMPs (but they cannot fix all signs of sun damage).

Cover Up

The majority of sun damage occurs not while you're at the beach or on a boating trip (when you are most likely slathered in sunscreen and wearing a hat); it happens during incidental activities. When waiting for your child at the school gate, driving your car, mowing the lawn, walking to the local shop, getting the mail — these kinds of activities account for two-thirds of your sunlight exposure. There is no better solution than to become a hat person and to wear a hat daily in order to protect your face.

This may feel weird at first, but you will soon find your comfort zone if you have a variety of hats to suit different occasions. Remember, it takes 21 days for new habits to stop feeling weird and to start feeling natural.

Consider buying three hats: one fashionable wide-brimmed hat or something to suit special occasions, one sports cap for exercise, and another hat to suit your daily outfits and activities. Hats, especially wide-brimmed ones, protect your face and, over the long term, will shave years off your skin's appearance.

For men, try on a felt fedora, a classic hat favored by celebrities such as Johnny Depp, or buy a straw fedora for the summer months. For casual outings or for outdoor work, nothing protects like a wide-brimmed straw hat, but a baseball cap will suffice.

Go for quality and personal appeal; a hat cannot save your face if it's sitting in the cupboard.

3. Barbecued Red Meats

If you want to eat a food that lengthens your lifespan and fights wrinkles, then don't throw a steak on the barbecue. According to a Food Habits in Later Life study of 2,000 people over the age of 70, the participants who frequently ate red meat had more skin wrinkling than those who

> If you want to eat a food that lengthens your lifespan and fights wrinkles, then don't throw a steak on the barbecue.

rarely consumed it. Animal-derived foods that are high in protein and fats, especially red meat and deli meats, are rich in wrinkle-promoting AGEs, and cooking causes new AGEs to form. In contrast, low-protein and low-fat foods, such as vegetables, fruits, and whole grains, contain relatively few AGEs, even after cooking.

> Wrinkles can be the least of your problems if you frequently eat meat. Frequent consumption of processed meats, such as bacon, hot dogs, and sausages, increases the risk of premature death by 20% — the same as if you smoked cigarettes.

The Research...

- Red meat contains high levels of AGEs before cooking, and these skin-sabotaging molecules increase during cooking.

- Of all the foods tested, steak cooked with olive oil contains the most AGEs, closely followed by plain cooked steak. Of the red meats, lamb contains slightly fewer AGEs.

- High intake of red meat is associated with higher levels of toxic nitrosamines, or N-nitroso compounds. And the amounts are comparable to those supplied in cigarette smoke. White meat, such as chicken and turkey, does not cause higher levels of N-nitroso compounds in humans.

- However, wrinkles can be the least of your problems if you frequently eat meat. A study of more than 120,000 people revealed that eating red meat — any amount and type — significantly increases the risk of premature death from cancer and heart disease. Researchers from the Harvard School of Public Health concluded that eating as little as 3 ounces (90 g) daily of unprocessed red meat increases the risk of death by 13%. Frequent consumption of processed meats, such as bacon, hot dogs, and sausages, increases the risk of premature death by 20% — the same as if you smoked cigarettes. The same study found that eating a handful of nuts instead of eating pork or a beef meal reduces the risk of dying by 19%. You are 14% safer if you substitute a red meat meal for one containing chicken or whole grains. If you swap lamb for legumes once a week, you are 10% better off, and choosing a fish dish instead of red meat reduces the risk of dying by 7%.

AGE Content in Protein Foods

N-(Carboxymethyl)lysine (CML) and methylglyoxal (MG) are two of the many types of AGEs that are associated with markers of disease and are elevated in patients with diabetes and kidney conditions. The following table lists a range of common protein foods and shows the content of AGEs of the CML variety only.

Content of Dietary AGEs in Protein Foods

Protein foods	Dietary AGEs in kU per 3½ oz (100 g)
Tuna, canned in water	452
Chicken, skinless breast, poached/cooked in casserole or soup with added lemon or tomato (acidic ingredient)	682
Tofu, raw	788
Chicken, skinless, parcel-baked with lemon	1047
Pork chop, pan-fried (7 minutes)	4752
Roast beef	6071
Steak, grilled or broiled	7478
Steak, pan-fried in olive oil	10,058

AGE Guide

For younger skin, reduce the amount of AGEs consumed as much as possible. As a guide, follow this recommended AGE intake:

- Foods considered low AGE contain 0 to 99 kU per 3½ oz (100 g)
- Low- to medium-AGE foods contain 100 to 999 kU per 3½ oz (100 g)
- High-AGE foods contain 1000 to 4999 kU per 3½ oz (100 g)
- Very-high-AGE foods contain more than 5000 kU per 3½ oz (100 g)

Halving

You can halve your daily intake of AGEs if you avoid red meat; prepare your chicken, tofu, or seafood (protein) meals by cooking with moist heat (such as by making soups, casseroles, and stews); and by ensuring you eat plenty of vegetables. Instead of frying, roasting, or grilling/broiling — all of which use high heat and greatly increase AGE production — try lemon poaching, parcel baking, or marinating protein foods, such as chicken and fish. These methods of cooking produce less than one-quarter of the dietary AGEs of frying.

4. Cheese (and Other Dairy Products)

> A week of eating ice cream every night is enough to cause visible changes in the skin.

Consuming dairy products increases your risk of wrinkles and sun damage, according to a study of 2,000 elderly Australians. The article, published in the *Journal of the American College of Nutrition*, revealed that the most wrinkled people frequently consumed butter, ice cream, or full-fat milk. A week of eating ice cream every night is enough to cause visible changes in the skin. It's no wonder: ice cream is packed with sugar, saturated fats, milk sugars, and additives.

Cheese	Dietary AGEs in kU per 3½ oz (100 g)
Cottage cheese, 1% fat	1453
Mozzarella, reduced fat	1677
Swiss cheese	4470
Brie	5597
Feta	8423
American cheese, white	8677
Parmesan, grated	16,900

The Research...

- The pasteurizing and homogenizing of dairy products, especially butter and cheeses, cause the formation of AGEs, which may partially explain why frequent dairy consumption is linked to wrinkle formation.

- Dairy consumption increases the risk of acne. Researchers suspect this could be due to the animal hormones and bioactive molecules found in milk products.

- High calcium intake from dairy products blocks the absorption of iron and zinc, which are essential minerals for collagen production in the skin.

- Cheeses, especially Parmesan, are rich in dietary AGEs. Fat-rich spreads, such as butter, margarine, and mayonnaise, are some of the richest sources of dietary AGEs.

For younger skin, avoid dairy products for at least 28 days. After 28 days, continue to avoid AGE-rich butter, margarine, and cheeses. Dairy alternatives are described on page 90.

5. Cigarettes

Smoking cigarettes can dramatically alter your physical appearance — the photos on cigarette packs are testament to that. Smokers with a history of heavy smoking are five times more likely to have wrinkles than non-smokers. However, as the advertisements say, every cigarette is doing you harm. Just one cigarette causes the constriction of blood vessels, which hampers blood flow to your skin. This leads to a dull complexion, wrinkled and dehydrated skin, and sores that won't heal — symptoms that are common with long-term smokers.

> Just one cigarette causes the constriction of blood vessels, which hampers blood flow to your skin. This leads to a dull complexion, wrinkled and dehydrated skin, and sores that won't heal.

The Research...

- Smoking decreases vitamin C levels in the body and it affects the body's ability to form healthy collagen in the skin.

- Tobacco contains high concentrations of wrinkle-promoting AGEs.

- Cigarette smoke induces matrix metalloproteinases (MMPs) in the skin, and MMPs play a role in skin aging.
- Smoking causes numerous dermatologic conditions, including poor wound healing, premature skin aging, squamous (scaly) cell cancers, psoriasis, and hair loss.
- A staggering 93.7% of sufferers of hidradenitis suppurativa — a chronic skin inflammation with blackheads, red bumps, and lesions that can enlarge and weep — are smokers or were previous smokers. For younger skin, enroll in a quit-smoking program today.

6. Lack of Exercise

> Exercise helps your body remove toxins and waste and it flushes the skin with lysozyme-rich sweat, which kills microbes that can cause skin inflammation.

Too busy to exercise? It could be costing you your looks and weakening the health of your whole body. Wounds heal slower in older adults who don't exercise, and the risk of skin infection is high when wound healing is delayed. Exercise helps your body remove toxins and waste and it flushes the skin with lysozyme-rich sweat, which kills microbes that can cause skin inflammation. Exercise also flushes the skin with nutrient-rich blood, giving your skin the building materials it needs for cell maintenance and renewal. What is most exciting about exercise and health is the effect it has on reducing glycation and AGE formation in the body.

As you age, hormone levels decline and your skin receives fewer nutrients and less oxygen as a result of hampered blood supply. This can leave the skin looking sallow — and inflammation, rashes, and other signs of aging are accelerated.

The Research...

- Frequent exercise reduces advanced glycation end product formation, so it has a protective effect against dietary AGEs and sugar-induced AGE formation.
- Exercise significantly speeds up wound healing in older adults.

- Frequent moderate exercise reduces inflammation, normalizes glucose metabolism, and improves renal function in patients with diabetes.

For younger skin, do some form of exercise every day to boost nutrient circulation to the skin. Exercise lessens the appearance of cellulite, and daily moderate- to high-impact exercise can prevent cellulite over the long term. Speak to a personal trainer if you are unsure of what the best forms of exercise are for your body type, level of health, and age.

7. Alcohol

Have you ever woken up after a night of drinking and found your face marked with an imprint from your sheets? Alcohol consumption severely dehydrates your skin and causes wrinkle formation, which can take hours to normalize. As you age, alcohol-induced wrinkles can occur on your face and chest, giving them an aged appearance.

Frequent alcohol consumption causes nutritional deficiencies — especially zinc, which is essential for collagen formation — and if left untreated, deficiencies can lead to a range of skin diseases, infections, and premature wrinkles.

According to Australia's Cancer Institute in New South Wales, we may have overestimated the health benefits of alcohol consumption. The heart-protective effects from consuming small amounts of alcohol only relate to people over the age of 45, and the health benefits of consuming alcohol outweigh its damaging effects only in mature women over the age of 65.

> The heart-protective effects from consuming small amounts of alcohol only relate to people over the age of 45, and the health benefits of consuming alcohol outweigh its damaging effects only in mature women over the age of 65.

The Research...

- People who frequently drink alcohol have elevated AGEs in the body.
- Alcohol consumption accelerates oxidative stress in the body (causing structural weaknesses, increased cell death, and tissue damage), which enhances the formation of AGEs and the stiffening of collagen in the skin.

- People who frequently drink alcohol can have multiple nutritional deficiencies, such as vitamin C and zinc deficiencies, which reduce skin elasticity and cause sagging skin.
- The elevation of AGEs in people who frequently drink alcohol might be caused, in part, by the deficiency of vitamins.

For younger skin, abstain from drinking alcohol for 28 days and limit alcohol consumption in the future.

8. Takeout and Fast Food

Trans fats cause one out of every five heart attacks in the United States.

Takeout and fast-food meals are a special treat for many Western families (some indulge more than others), but is your Friday fish 'n' chips night ruining your skin? Fast-food outlets use oils that are heated repeatedly, and these oils change form when cooked at high temperatures. They become harmful trans fats, which behave like saturated fats in the body. It is estimated that trans fats cause one out of

Amount of AGEs in Various Fast Foods

Takeout and fast foods	Dietary AGEs in kU per 3½ oz (100 g) unless otherwise specified
Soy burger	55
French fries	1522
Eggs (2), fried in margarine	2749
Potato chips	2883
Tofu, fried/sautéed	4723
Cheese melt, toasted, open-faced	5679
Chicken nuggets (3 oz/90 g)	8627
2 slices pizza (6 oz/175 g)	12,285
Beef hamburger (7½ oz/216 g)	16,850

every five heart attacks in the United States, according to the Harvard School of Public Health. Trans fats cause inflammation and increase the risk of heart disease, obesity, strokes, diabetes, and high cholesterol.

Fried foods that are cooked with quality heat-resistant oils are less prone to trans fats, but they pose a different problem: they are rich in AGEs (anything over 1000 kU per $3\frac{1}{2}$ ounce/100 g is considered high or very high), which attack skin collagen, decreasing skin elasticity.

Cooking Methods

Although poaching, steaming, and boiling foods are methods that use lower heat (up to 200°F/100°C), other cooking methods use temperatures that greatly increase AGE formation in foods:

- Grilling/broiling: 425°F (220°C)
- Deep-frying: 350°F (180°C)
- Roasting: 350°F (180°C)
- Oven-frying: 450°F (230°C)

The searing heat used in baking and oven-frying causes browning, and this increases AGEs formation in foods, especially in protein- and fat-rich foods. Fried foods from fast-foods outlets — especially oven-fried foods, such as chicken nuggets and pizza — are incredibly rich in AGEs and they are literally aging you.

For younger skin, you know what to do: avoid fast foods and use gentler cooking methods, such as poaching, boiling, stewing, soup-making, and steaming — and don't forget raw foods, which are the lowest in AGEs.

> Fried foods from fast-foods outlets — especially oven-fried foods, such as chicken nuggets and pizza — are incredibly rich in AGEs and they are literally aging you.

FAQ

Q. Will I have to avoid pan-frying or baking foods during the 28 days?

A. You do not need to avoid these cooking methods. The recipe section will show you how to fry and bake foods in a slightly different way that minimizes AGE formation during cooking.

9. Burnt Toast

A piece of toast or a bowl of cereal might be standard breakfast food, but is breaking the fast with crispy processed foods damaging your skin? Buttered slices of toast contain AGEs that increase in density with increased toasting, so you might want to turn down the setting on your toaster and opt for healthier spreads. It is not just toast that is a problem: processed breakfast cereals containing toasted flakes, crispy biscuits, or puffed grains contain their share of AGEs, too.

Carbohydrate foods	Dietary AGEs in kU per 3½ oz (100 g) unless otherwise specified
White rice, boiled	9
Oatmeal, cooked (porridge)	14
Bran flakes	33
2 slices whole wheat bread (3½ oz/100 g), untoasted (no butter or margarine)	53
2 slices whole wheat bread (3½ oz/100 g), toasted	137
White pita, toasted	607
Corn chips (average of two brands)	886
Croissant	1113
Pretzel sticks	1600
Doughnut, chocolate iced	1803
Rice Krispies breakfast cereal	2000
Toasted cereal bar	2143
2 slices white bread, toasted (2 oz/60 g), with butter (⅓ oz/10 g)	2712
Waffle, toasted	2870
Cookie, biscotti	3220

Compared with protein foods, such as red meat, butter, and fast foods, carbohydrates contain fewer dietary AGEs. However, carbohydrate foods cause an AGE problem another way: they supply glucose and cause it to spike in the blood, which can set off a glycation reaction that can lead to irreversible AGE formation.

The Research...

- Commercial breakfast cereals, toast, crackers, and cookies that have been baked until crispy contain 10 times the amount of dietary AGEs compared to untoasted bread (without butter or margarine).

- Whole-grain breads contain up to 70% fewer AGEs than processed white bread.

- Whole grains don't generally increase AGEs in the body unless they have been toasted, cooked to a crisp, or buttered.

- Untoasted breakfast cereals, such as rolled oats or porridge, reduce the risk of heart disease and premature death; the consumption of refined breakfast cereals does not have the same protective effect.

> For younger skin, opt for low-GI whole-grain foods.

For younger skin, opt for low-GI whole-grain foods, such as oats, untoasted muesli, porridge, quinoa, basmati rice, whole wheat pasta (such as spelt pasta), or whole-grain spelt bread. And keep the toaster setting on Low.

10. Deli Meats

Deli meats, including ham, salami, sausages, and bacon, may be rich in flavor, but they are also rich sources of advanced glycation end products. Deli meats largely owe their flavors to saturated fats, artificial flavor enhancers, and smoking methods that cause the AGE content to skyrocket. There is plenty of research to suggest that deli meats are not only harmful to your skin, but may also shorten your lifespan. For younger skin, swap AGE-rich deli meats for fresh foods cooked on low heat.

The Research...

- Researchers from the Harvard School of Public Health found that the frequent consumption of processed meats, such as bacon, hot dogs, and sausages, increases the risk of premature death by 20% — the same as if you smoked cigarettes.

- Processed meats contain very high levels of AGEs and toxic nitrosamines, which increase the risk of cancer, heart disease, and diabetes.

Deli meats	Dietary AGEs in kU per 3½ oz (100 g) unless otherwise specified
Salmon, smoked	572
Deli ham, smoked	2349
Turkey breast, smoked, seared	6013
Bacon, microwaved for 3 minutes	9022
2 pork sausages (6 oz/175 g), microwaved for 1 minute	10,698
2 strips of bacon (2 oz/50 g), pan-fried	11,000
2 beef hot dogs (6 oz/175 g), boiled for 5 minutes	13,472
2 beef hot dogs (6 oz/175 g), grilled or broiled for 5 minutes	20,286

11. Butter and Margarine

The types of fats you eat can show on your face — consume too many saturated fats, from foods such as butter and red meat, and you can either develop pimples or get dry, prematurely aged skin (depending on your genetics, you could end up with both). Margarines are problematic as well, because they contain varying levels of polyunsaturated and monounsaturated oils that have been tampered with in order to make them solid and spreadable. Some brands contain trans fat, which behaves like saturated fat in the body. Margarines also contain preservatives and other artificial additives. They are rich sources of omega-6 fatty acids, which Western populations consume in abundance. Research shows that families who frequently use margarine are more likely to have children who develop eczema by the age of 2. Both butter and margarine are rich sources of dietary AGEs and both can age your skin.

> Research shows that families who frequently use margarine are more likely to have children who develop eczema by the age of 2.

The Research...

- Butter and margarine top the AGE-rich list, closely followed by processed or "light" olive oil.
- Olive oil that is cold-pressed is far lower in AGEs because it has not been heated during the manufacturing process.
- Avocado, which is unprocessed and rich in monounsaturated fat, is far lower in AGEs than other fat-rich spreads.

Fats, spreads	Dietary AGEs in kU per $\frac{1}{3}$ oz (10 g)
Avocado	157
Mayonnaise	940
Extra virgin olive oil, cold-pressed	1004
Olive oil, processed with heat	1200
Margarine	1752
Butter	2648

12. Overeating

Research shows that overweight people have elevated AGEs in their blood. Overeating (and under-exercising) can not only greatly increase the amount of AGEs you accumulate in your body, this pattern can also shorten your lifespan and lead to all sorts of health problems, including heart disease and diabetes. The modern Western diet is partly to blame, because diets rich in sugar and artificial sweeteners can trigger overeating, and excess consumption of red meat and fried foods is favored.

The Research...

- High-protein diets greatly increase the burden of AGEs in the body and can cause kidney damage.
- Elevated blood levels of AGEs in obese and overweight adults can be successfully reduced by a low-calorie diet.
- If you reduce your dietary intake of AGEs by 50%, you can reduce levels of oxidative stress and lessen deterioration of insulin sensitivity and kidney function as you age.

If you are unsure if you are within a healthy weight range, ask your doctor.

For younger skin, if you are obese or overweight, a low-calorie diet is recommended for weight loss, but it is not necessary if you are within the healthy weight range for your height.

Swapping Foods

If you substitute higher-AGEs foods with lower ones, you can improve the quality of your skin.

Swap this	For that
Red meat	Skinless chicken, marinated with lemon
Pork/bacon/ham	Marinated fish or tofu
Deli meats	Raw nuts and seeds
Sausages	Seafood or beans
Beef, ground	Turkey, ground, cooked with liquids or tomato
Cow's milk	Non-dairy milks (such as organic soy milk)
Butter/margarine	Hummus dip or avocado
Cheese	Raw nuts and seeds
Processed breakfast cereal	Rolled oats or porridge (oat or quinoa)

Recap

- Reduce the amount of sugars consumed in your diet.
- Your face is your fortune — protect it with a hat.
- Abstain from drinking alcohol for 28 days.
- Don't burn your toast.
- Reduce your intake of dietary AGEs by reducing your intake of solid fats (butter and margarine), beef and other fatty meats, dairy products, and fried foods, and by increasing your consumption of fish, legumes, vegetables, fruits, and whole grains.
- Halve the amount of AGEs by changing the way you prepare food, by using medium- to low-heat cooking methods.
- Instead of frying, roasting, or grilling, use low-AGE cooking methods, such as poaching, boiling, and steaming, and make soups, curries, stews, and casseroles.

FAQ

Q. How much should I eat?

A. Eat three main meals and a couple of snacks each day. Avoid skipping meals, because this can mess with your blood sugar levels and promote fatigue and sugar cravings (and sugar bingeing, which is bad for your skin). Here are some guidelines:

Breakfast

Your serving size can vary, but it is important to eat something healthy that fills you up so you have enough energy to get you through until lunch. The menus, beginning on page 153, will give you some healthy choices.

Lunch and dinner

Fill half your plate with vegetables, one-quarter with a quality protein, such as chicken, fish, or legumes, and the other quarter with quality carbohydrates, such as sweet potato, basmati rice, quinoa, or spelt. If you want to avoid carbohydrates at night, you can consume extra vegetables in place of grains with your dinner.

How much food should go on your plate?

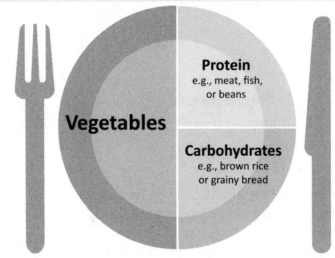

Dessert

Favor antioxidant-rich fruits, such as guava, banana, papaya, or berries of any kind (frozen mixed berries are great), or try the smoothie recipes, which start on page 173.

Don't go hungry. There are plenty of delicious recipes and foods to choose from, so stock the fridge with healthy ingredients before you begin the 28-day program. The menus, which begin on page 153, and the shopping list, on page 159, will show you what to do.

FAQ

Q. How much coffee and tea can I drink?

A. Coffee contains beans that have been roasted, making coffee a source of AGEs, but (thankfully) the beans have not been processed enough to put coffee in the Dirty Dozen. Coffee does contain caffeine, however, so I recommend you limit coffee intake to 1 or 2 cups (250 to 500 mL) daily (and avoid coffee that has been brewing in a pot for hours — it is rich in AGEs).

Or opt for black tea and herbal teas; they are practically AGE-free. Naturally caffeine-free herbal teas, such as ginger, peppermint, and lemon, are excellent choices. Favor herbal teas or chai tea (leaf variety, not the powder) because they contain alkalizing ginger, cinnamon, and cloves, so they have a balance of acid and alkaline ingredients.

Keep in mind that most teas, especially black tea, contain tannins that bind to iron; this can cause iron deficiency if you frequently drink teas with your meals or close to mealtimes.

If you choose to drink tea, sip it in between meals and ensure you are consuming enough iron for good health. See iron information on page 106. If you drink a coffee or tea during the 28-day program, I suggest that you exercise afterward, drink a vegetable juice, or eat a salad to restore the acid–alkaline balance to your diet.

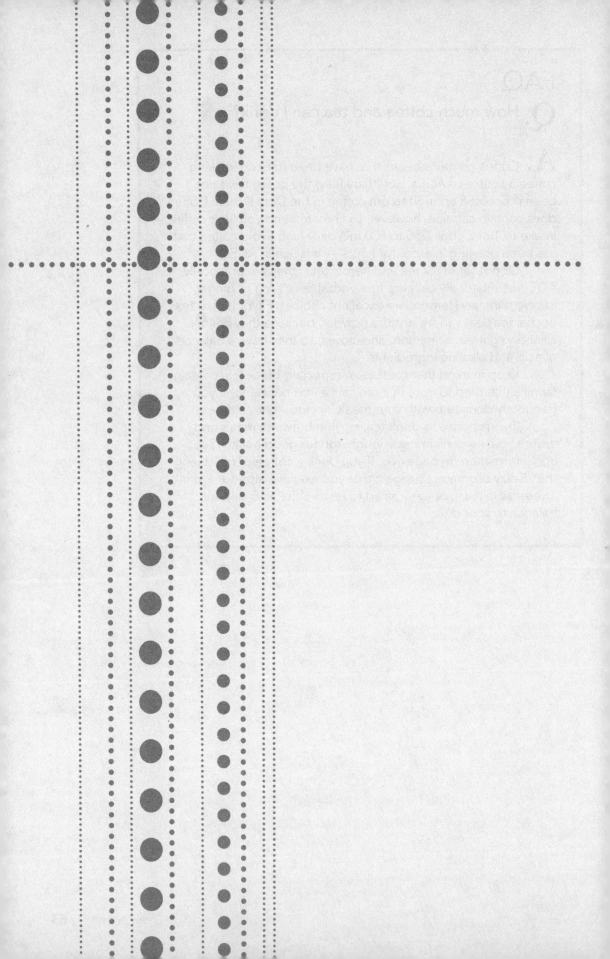

Chapter 4

Top 12 Foods for Younger Skin

· ·

The best weapon against skin aging is your fork. Eating the right foods supplies your skin with the nutrients it needs to produce new collagen, fight AGEs, and look healthier and younger. The top 12 anti-AGE foods can help you create younger skin and a healthy body, and the menu plans later in the book will show you how to incorporate them into your daily diet. Here are the top 12 anti-AGE foods for younger skin, with recommended recipes.

1. Dark Leafy Greens

Dark green salad leaves are highly alkalizing and beneficial for the skin thanks to their rich chlorophyll content. Dark leafy greens also deliver more nutrients for fewer calories than other salad greens, and the calcium in kale and watercress is easy for the body to absorb. Greens contain antioxidants, folate, magnesium, calcium, beta-carotene, vitamin C, B-group vitamins, potassium, and cancer-protective phytonutrients, plus they are gluten-free and low on the glycemic index. Varieties include Chinese greens, kale, dandelion greens, silver beet, spinach, chicory, beet greens, mustard greens, arugula, watercress, and baby spinach.

> Dark green salad leaves are highly alkalizing and beneficial for the skin thanks to their rich chlorophyll content.

   Recommended recipes: Green Glow Juice (page 177), Scrambled Eggs with Watercress (page 171), Guava and Arugula Salad (page 192), and Watercress Soup (page 186).

Anthocyanins

Anthocyanins are powerful antioxidant flavonoids. They are also nature's sunscreen — a protective pigment giving fruits, vegetables, and some grains their purple, blue, red, or black hues. Think: eggplant, cherries, blueberries, pomegranates, and black rice (purple corn and purple carrots, too). There are more than 300 types of anthocyanins found in nature. Prehistoric and traditional

Anti-Aging Effects of Anthocyanins

- Protect blood vessels from oxidative damage
- Can reduce high blood sugar levels in people with diabetes
- Help neutralize enzymes that can destroy connective tissue in the skin
- Can repair damaged proteins in blood vessel walls, and their anti-inflammatory properties activate the production of type II collagen
- Block metalloproteinases (MMP-1, MMP-9), which degrade collagen and elastic fibers and play a role in skin aging
- Offer mild UV protection
- Have anticancer properties, and purple pigmented foods, such as eggplant, may be beneficial for those undergoing cancer treatment and chemotherapy
- Anti-inflammatory properties help to protect against glycation and AGE formation

diets were abundant in berries and other anthocyanin-rich foods, but modern Western diets are relatively low in them.

A German study found that people with diabetes who took a supplement of 600 mg of anthocyanins daily for 2 months had a reduction in abnormal collagen production.

2. Red Quinoa

Quinoa (pronounced *keen-wah*) is a healthy gluten-free seed and, although a seed, it was referred to by the ancient Incas as the mother of all grains. It is rich in carbohydrates, but also abundant in antioxidants, folate, iron, magnesium, zinc, dietary fiber, and protein. Both red quinoa and the black variety are lower in carbohydrates than white quinoa and owe their rich color to anthocyanins. As with many carbohydrate-rich foods, quinoa can affect your blood sugar levels (white quinoa has a higher glycemic index, but the darker varieties have a lower GI). Favor red quinoa and eat it with cinnamon, which will help keep your blood sugar levels steady.

> Favor red quinoa and eat it with cinnamon, which will help keep your blood sugar levels steady.

You can use quinoa as an alternative to rice: just boil it with vegetable stock for 20 minutes. Recommended recipes: Quinoa and Pomegranate Salad (page 196), Oregano Chicken Skewers (page 208), or Quinoa Porridge (page 168). See also How to Cook Quinoa, page 209.

3. Black Sesame Seeds

Black sesame seeds are similar to the white variety, except the black ones are not hulled and are far more nutritious. The black seeds taste as if they are toasted, so you don't have to fry them to get that delicious nutty flavor. They are rich in protective anthocyanins, which give the seeds their blackened hue. They are also a source of protein, magnesium, and zinc, which are essential for healthy skin and new collagen formation. Sprinkle some black sesame seeds onto salads or rice dishes.

Recommended recipes: Sushi Rolls with Black Sesame (page 202), Mango and Black Sesame Salad (page 193), Beet and Carrot Salad (page 194), Guava and Arugula Salad (page 192), and Sweet Potato Salad (page 195).

4. Blueberries

Berries contain anthocyanins, which give blueberries their dark purple pigment. The other antioxidants present in this superfood are resveratrol, vitamin C, and vitamin E, which work together to give blueberries their strong anti-glycation properties. Research shows the unique range of phenolic compounds in berries significantly reduce the generation of harmful AGEs. There is promising research showing that resveratrol has the ability to inhibit chemical-induced skin cancers, so this particular antioxidant is of great interest to researchers in anti-aging and skin-care fields.

It's easy to grow your own blueberries — first check to see if the climate is suitable in your area. The homegrown, fresh varieties are even more delicious than the store-bought varieties.

Recommended recipes: blueberries make a great addition to Omega Muesli (page 166), Berry Porridge (page 167), and desserts, or add frozen blueberries to Moisture Boost Smoothie (page 174).

5. Pomegranate

Ellagic acid is an important flavonoid antioxidant found in pomegranates, blackberries, cranberries, pecans, raspberries, strawberries, grapes, and walnuts.

Pomegranate is an exotic red fruit and an important source of antioxidants, including anthocyanins and vitamin C. The bioflavonoid antioxidants present in pomegranate seeds help to protect against free radical production and inflammation, which can damage cells. Commercially prepared pomegranate juice (which has a little of the rind tannins present) has an antioxidant activity three times greater than that of green tea or red wine. Fresh-squeezed pomegranate juice has twice the antioxidant activity.

Ellagic acid is an important flavonoid antioxidant found in pomegranates, blackberries, cranberries, pecans, raspberries, strawberries, grapes, and walnuts. Studies show that ellagic acid prevents AGE formation and that this anti-glycating effect could help control AGE-mediated diabetic symptoms and AGE-related eyesight problems. Pomegranate also contains gallic acid, which inhibits the accumulation of advanced glycation end products and protects collagen.

Recommended recipes: pomegranate seeds are best eaten by adding them to salads, such as Quinoa and Pomegranate Salad (page 196), or drink half a cup (125 mL) of commercial pure pomegranate juice (no added sugar). For tips on how to remove the seeds from a pomegranate, see How to Choose and Seed a Pomegranate on page 197.

6. Red Onion

Most onions, including red onion, are rich in quercetin, a potent antioxidant that protects against oxidative damage and AGE formation. Red onion has the added benefit of containing colored anthocyanins that lower blood sugar and activate the production of collagen in the skin. Red onions have strong antifungal, anti-inflammatory, and antibacterial properties thanks to allicin, an organic sulfur compound that gives onions their unique taste and smell.

Korean researchers tested 25 common plants and found that red onion had the most potent array of antioxidants and anti-glycation activity, which protects against AGE formation in the skin. Red onions have antidiabetic properties; consuming 3½ ounces (100 g) of raw red onion reduces blood glucose levels to within a healthy range. Simply add any amount of raw or cooked red onion to soups, casseroles, and salads to make an anti-AGE meal.

Recommended recipes: Anti-Aging Broth (page 184), Shiitake Vegetable Soup (page 188), Spiced Sweet Potato Soup (page 187), and Moroccan Lemon Chicken (page 207).

> Red onions have strong antifungal, anti-inflammatory, and antibacterial properties thanks to allicin, an organic sulfur compound that gives onions their unique taste and smell.

FAQ

Q. Do I really need to drink lots of water?

A. Yes. Drink 8 glasses of hydrating liquids daily, including filtered water, herbal teas, and fresh vegetable juices.

7. Red Guava

Guavas contain ellagic acid and anthocyanins, which offer strong antioxidant protection and inhibit the formation of advanced glycation end products.

Guava is one of the most nutritious fruits, with up to 300 mg of vitamin C per 3½ ounces (100 g) — six times more vitamin C than oranges — and it is a rich source of lycopene, which helps to protect the skin from sun damage and skin cancer. Guavas contain ellagic acid and anthocyanins, which offer strong antioxidant protection and inhibit the formation of advanced glycation end products. The fruit has the added benefit of lowering blood sugar.

Rich in gallic acid and quercetin, guava leaf extract (a herbal extract) strongly inhibits high blood sugar and the formation of AGEs. The active compounds in guava also help to restore anti-aging antioxidant enzymes, including superoxide dismutase (SOD) and glutathione peroxidase, making guava a super anti-aging fruit.

Recommended recipes: Papaya Cups with Lime and Guava (page 226) and Guava and Arugula Salad (page 192). Or have them as a snack: the skin is edible — just wash them and remove the seeds. If guava is not in season, buy cherries.

8. Yellow Curry Powder

Yellow curry powder contains a range of powerful spices that protect your skin from AGE-related damage. Turmeric gives curry its yellow-orange color thanks to the presence of curcumin. Curcumin has been widely researched because it has an exciting spectrum of therapeutic activities, including anti-inflammatory, antioxidant, anticancer, antibacterial, antifungal, antiviral, and blood-thinning properties. In research studies, curcumin improves collagen formation and accelerates wound healing; it inhibits AGE formation and prevents collagen cross-linking and damage.

Cumin seeds are typically used in the form of ground cumin to create a delicious mild-flavored curry. Cumin has been touted as an antidiabetic spice. It is almost as potent as cinnamon when it comes to lowering blood sugar levels.

Cumin is also capable of reducing oxidative stress and inhibiting AGE formation and the cross-linking of proteins, making it a wonderful addition to any anti-aging diet.

Ginger can be consumed as fresh gingerroot or ground ginger. It is another common curry spice that inhibits glycation, and it has an anti-inflammatory effect on the skin. Ginger also boosts levels of the important anti-aging enzymes glutathione (GSH) and superoxide dismutase (SOD), which play a role in longevity and younger skin.

Recommended recipes: Eggplant and Cauliflower Curry (page 200), Winter Spiced Dal (page 201), Curry Naan Bread (variation, page 214), Moroccan Lemon Chicken (page 207), and Steamed Chicken and Mint Meatballs (page 210).

9. Cloves

According to research studies, of all the herbs and spices, cloves are the best at preventing AGE formation. Cloves are unopened flower buds and have been highly prized since ancient times. Cloves were used to sweeten the breath of Chinese emperors. Cloves' medicinal properties are antifungal, antiviral, anti-inflammatory, antimicrobial, antidiabetic, and antithrombotic. According to research studies, a drop of clove oil has antioxidants 400 times more powerful than blueberries. Eugenol, the key ingredient in cloves, reduces inflammation by blocking series 2 prostaglandin formation.

> Clove tea is beneficial for eliminating intestinal worms, *Candida albicans*, and other parasites — but be warned, a high dose of clove can cause a temporary bowel flushing effect.

Clove tea is beneficial for eliminating intestinal worms, *Candida albicans*, and other parasites — but be warned, a high dose of clove can cause a temporary bowel flushing effect, which helps with the elimination process. Cloves are best used in curries in the form of garam masala, a popular spice mix made from ground cloves, cinnamon, cumin, black pepper, and cardamom. Cloves are often used in chai tea — favor the leaf or tea bag varieties (not powdered chai, which is rich in sugar and powdered dairy milk).

Recommended recipes: Chai Tea with Clove (page 180), Watercress Soup (page 186), Eggplant and Cauliflower Curry (page 200), and Moroccan Lemon Chicken (page 207).

You can confidently enjoy quality whole-grain carbs in moderation if you add a dash of cinnamon to the meal.

10. Cinnamon

Cinnamon is the second-best spice (after cloves) at inhibiting AGE formation. And it has the added benefit of containing protective phytochemicals, such as cinnamaldehyde, which reduces blood sugar levels, promotes satiety (so you're less likely to overeat), and lowers LDL ("bad") cholesterol. What is most exciting and useful about cinnamon is its potent ability to slow the absorption of carbohydrates in the bowel, so your body needs less insulin to control blood sugar, making cinnamon a super anti-aging spice. This is good news because it means you can confidently enjoy quality whole-grain carbs in moderation if you add a dash of cinnamon to the meal.

Recommended recipes: Omega Muesli (page 166), Quinoa Porridge (page 168), Moisture Boost Smoothie (page 174), Spelt Flatbread (page 214), Eggplant and Cauliflower Curry (page 200), Oregano Chicken Skewers (page 208), and Shiitake Vegetable Casserole (page 199).

Buying Cinnamon: What to Look For

All types of cinnamon are fine to use in moderation, but Ceylon cinnamon is the top choice. Chinese cinnamon and cassia cinnamon — the most common varieties used in ground or powdered cinnamon — are rich in coumarin, which can be toxic in very high doses but fine to consume in small amounts, such as those recommended in cooking. If you like to use a lot of cinnamon, look for Ceylon cinnamon, which is usually only available as whole cinnamon sticks, known as quills. When ground at home, Ceylon cinnamon is sweeter tasting and more aromatic than the other varieties. Spotting authentic Ceylon cinnamon is easy — the bark is softer and thinner than other types of cinnamon, and Ceylon cinnamon quills also roll up in one direction, whereas other types of cinnamon bark roll from both directions and meet in the center like a scroll. Ceylon cinnamon is easy to break apart, so you can grind it in a seed or coffee grinder or use a mortar and pestle to make it into lovely fragrant ground cinnamon.

However, any form of cinnamon is better than none, so buy what you can. Add it to breakfast cereals, porridge, smoothies, and quinoa recipes, or use the spice mix garam masala in curries (because it contains both cinnamon and cloves).

11. Lemons and Limes

Lemons and limes are two of the best fruits for younger skin. Lemons and limes are not only highly alkalizing, they also supply vitamin C. When they are added to meals, they significantly reduce AGE formation. Lemons and limes are acidic before digestion, but once in the body, they become highly alkalizing and great for the skin.

If you like eating protein foods, such as chicken or fish, coat the protein in a marinade that includes lemon or lime juice to reduce AGEs formation during cooking.

Recommended recipes: Tamari, Lycopene and Lemon Marinade (page 220), Ginger and Lime Dipping Sauce (page 222), Flaxseed Lemon Drink (page 175), Parcel-Baked Fish (page 204), and Steamed Fish with Coconut and Lime Marinade (page 206).

> Lemons and limes are acidic before digestion, but once in the body, they become highly alkalizing and great for the skin.

FAQ

Q. What does it mean when foods are said to be "acid-forming" or "highly alkalizing"?

A. This refers to how a food affects your pH level. Your food does more than stop the hunger pangs and boost your energy; once your meal is digested, it releases either an acid or an alkaline base into your bloodstream. To be healthy, your blood needs to be slightly alkaline, at a pH between 7.35 and 7.45, and your body will do all it can to keep the blood within these limits. For example, if you eat a lot of acid-forming foods and have high stress in your life (which promotes acid), your body will store some of the acids in your tissues, rob some calcium (which is alkaline) from your bones, and secrete acid through the kidneys in order to keep the blood at the correct pH level. So to protect your skin tissues and kidneys from damage, and your bones from calcium loss, it pays to have plenty of alkalizing foods in your diet — and fewer (or a balance) of the acidifying ones.

Over the long term, a diet rich in highly acid-forming foods (beef, corn, white flour, and white sugar, to name a few) will cause, among other issues, low-grade metabolic acidosis, which causes a decline in kidney function as you age. It can also cause a loss of bone density. Keeping your diet in acid–alkaline

continued, next page

balance (a balance of alkalizing vegetables and healthy acid-forming foods, such as fish, beans, and whole grains) promotes strong bones and lightens the acid burden your kidneys have to deal with each day. Alkalizing foods also promote younger skin because they aid the removal of toxins from the body. When enough alkalizing foods are consumed in the diet, the urine pH can exceed an alkaline reading of 7.5 and alkalization occurs. This enhances the liver's ability to detoxify chemicals, including preservatives, amines, food colorings, MSG, and salicylates. For example, when the urine pH exceeds 7.5, three times the amount of salicylates are deactivated and removed from the body via the urine. This is especially useful if you have salicylate and chemical sensitivities because it decreases the occurrence of negative reactions to foods over time, thereby allowing you to eat a more varied diet. Alkalizing foods also thin the blood, so blood flow to the skin is improved, giving your skin a healthy glow.

It is easy to check if your diet is acid–alkaline balanced by testing the pH of your saliva or urine using litmus paper. The reading will change throughout the day depending on what you eat and drink, and stress can also greatly increase acid in the body, so remember to relax and take care of your mental health, too.

There is much debate as to what foods are alkalizing, and often most fruits and some grains are listed as alkalizing, which is untrue — most fruits and all grains are acid-forming, but you can still enjoy them when balanced with alkalizing foods.

Recommended foods: foods that are alkalizing include raw almonds, pretty much all vegetables (not cooked spinach, but raw spinach is highly alkalizing), and a few fruits, such as lemons, limes, avocado, raw tomato, and bananas, which are listed on the charts on pages 76–79. The recipes in this book show you how to prepare and serve tasty acid–alkaline-balanced meals.

12. Kumato

Kumato, a sweet and semi-black tomato, possesses an important skin nutrient that regular tomatoes do not — it is rich in AGE-reducing anthocyanins, which give the blackened appearance to the skin. Kumatoes are also rich in vitamin C and beta-carotene, which are known to fight some forms of cancer and heart disease.

Like traditional tomatoes, Kumato tomatoes are rich in lycopene, an important red carotenoid. Lycopene builds up in the skin in direct proportion to how much lycopene is in your diet, and it has a mild sunscreen effect within the skin. Lycopene also helps the body remove toxins and carcinogens (cancer-causing substances) because it enhances phase I and II liver detoxification reactions, and it has anticancer and antioxidant properties, too. Raw tomato is a rich source of lycopene, but after cooking, the lycopene content markedly increases. Tomatoes are a rich source of flavonoids, including quercetin, which has strong anti-inflammatory and antioxidant properties that are wonderful for the skin.

If you cannot find Kumatoes, look for Black Russian, plum (Roma), vine-ripened, or grape tomatoes.

Recommended recipes: Guava and Arugula Salad (page 192), Mango and Black Sesame Salad (page 193), and Oregano Chicken Skewers (page 208).

> Raw tomato is a rich source of lycopene, but after cooking, the lycopene content markedly increases.

Recap

- Eat 1 cup (250 mL) of purple foods each day — such as purple salad leaves, purple kale, blueberries, red onion, red cabbage, eggplant, purple broccoli, or purple carrots — to encourage collagen production and reduce AGE formation.

- Eat 1/2 cup (125 mL) of red foods daily — including red quinoa, tomato, red bell pepper, pomegranate, and guava — this is important to ensure you consume enough vitamin C for collagen production.

- Eat a serving of black foods several times weekly, such as 1 teaspoon (5 mL) black sesame seeds, 1/2 cup (125 mL) black quinoa or black rice, or a handful of Kumatoes or blackberries. Note that some black foods are not black due to anthocyanins — for example, black pasta is dyed with squid ink and does not contain anthocyanins.

- Add spices to your daily diet, such as 1 tablespoon (15 mL) yellow curry powder to make a curry; make black tea special by adding a slice of fresh ginger and a clove; and control blood sugar with a small sprinkle of cinnamon on oats or added to smoothies, curries, and casseroles.

- Use fresh lemon and lime in your cooking because they reduce AGE formation and supply vitamin C for collagen support.

Acid–Alkaline Food Charts

The following charts list alkalizing and acidifying products. They also show the main natural and artificial chemicals present, for those who have sensitivities.

Symbols and Abbreviations

MSG natural or artificial flavor enhancer
GI food with a high glycemic index (use cinnamon with it!)
G contains gluten
P may contain preservatives and/or artificial sweeteners/flavors/colors
Ω a good source of omega-3 fatty acids (eat fish three times a week, plus flax seeds and flaxseed oil daily, if no allergy)

Strongly Alkalizing	Alkalizing	Acidifying	Strongly Acidifying
Beverages			
Anti-Aging Broth (page 184)	Almond Milk (page 172) or store-bought almond milk	Beer	Alcohol
Cucumber and Mint Juice (page 176)	Herbal teas	Carob powder	Black tea
Flaxseed Lemon Drink (page 175)	Mineral water, non-carbonated, unflavored	Fruit juice	Cocoa, hot chocolate (P)
Green detox powder	Moisture Boost Smoothie (page 174)	Green tea	Coffee (P)
Green Glow Juice (page 177)	Vegetable juice, packaged (MSG)	Milk, dairy, processed	Cordial (P)
Liquid chlorophyll; Green Water (page 182)	Water, plain-filtered or from a spring	Mineral water, carbonated, no flavor	Dried soup mixes (MSG, P)
Purple Carrot Juice (page 178)		Rice milk, plain (GI)	Soft drinks (sodas), flavored (P)
Vegetable juice, fresh		Soy milk, plain	Water, tap
Wheatgrass juice		Tomato juice (MSG)	
Fruits			
Strongly Alkalizing	Alkalizing	Acidifying	Strongly Acidifying
Grapefruit	Apricots, dried	Apples, raw	Black currants
Lemons	Avocados	Apricots, raw	Blackthorn berries
Limes	Bananas, dried (P)	Blueberries, raw	Kiwifruit
	Bananas, raw	Cherries, raw	Mandarin oranges
	Dates, dried (GI)	Dried fruits (maybe MSG)	Mulberries
	Raisins (MSG)	Figs, fresh and dried	Nectarines
	Tomatoes, raw (MSG)	Grapes (MSG)	Oranges
	Mangos, fresh and dried		Pineapples

Fruits *(continued)*

Strongly Alkalizing	Alkalizing	Acidifying	Strongly Acidifying
	Papayas		
	Pears		
	Persimmons		
	Plums (MSG)		
	Pomegranates		
	Prunes (MSG)		
	Raspberries		
	Strawberries		
	Tomatoes, cooked (MSG)		
	Watermelon		

Vegetables

Strongly Alkalizing	Alkalizing	Acidifying	Strongly Acidifying
Alfalfa sprouts	Artichokes	Bamboo shoots	Pickled cucumbers
Arugula	Asparagus	Peas, fresh (MSG)	Pickled vegetables (in vinegar)
Beet greens, raw	Bell peppers	Peas, dried	
Beets, raw (GI)	Brussels sprouts		
Broccoli (MSG)	Cabbage		
Cucumber	Carrots		
Dandelion greens	Cauliflower		
Dark leafy greens, raw	Celery		
Kale, raw	Chard, cooked (MSG)		
Lentil sprouts	Chicory		
Mung bean sprouts	Chinese greens		
Parsley	Eggplant		
Snow pea sprouts	Garlic		
Spinach, raw (MSG)	Green beans		
Watercress	Green onions		
	Leeks		
	Lettuce		
	Mushrooms (MSG)		
	Olives		
	Onions		
	Pumpkin		
	Snow peas		
	Spinach, cooked		
	Summer squash		
	Turnips		
	Winter squash		
	Zucchini		

Carbohydrates: Potatoes, Grains, Flours, and Breads

Strongly Alkalizing	Alkalizing	Acidifying	Strongly Acidifying
	Potatoes, new Potatoes, red (GI) Potatoes, white (GI) Sprouted grains Sprouted bread (G) Sweet potatoes	Barley (G) Bread, pumpernickel (G) Bread, spelt sourdough (G) Bread, whole wheat (G) Bread, whole-grain (G) Buckwheat Oats, rolled (G) Pasta, spelt (G) Quinoa Rice milk, plain (GI) Rice, brown Rye flour (G) Soy flour	All-purpose flour (GI, G) Bread, white (GI, G) Bread, yeast (G) Corn Corn tortillas, chips, tacos Corn flakes cereal (GI) Cornstarch (GI) Millet (GI) Pasta, white wheat (G) Polenta (GI) Processed wheat cereals (GI, G) Rice, basmati Rice, white jasmine (GI)

Nuts, Seeds, Oils, and Fats

Strongly Alkalizing	Alkalizing	Acidifying	Strongly Acidifying
	Almonds Brazil nuts Butter, pure (no additives to soften) Coconut oil Cold-pressed oils (unrefined, unheated) Extra virgin olive oil Flax seeds Flaxseed oil	Cashews, roasted Coconut Cold-pressed oils (heated) Safflower oil Sunflower oil Sesame seeds	Butter, heated Hazelnuts Hydrogenated fats Lard Margarine (P) Peanut oil Peanuts Pecans Pistachios Pumpkin seeds Sunflower seeds Walnuts

Condiments, Sweeteners, Sweets, Salt, and Spices

Strongly Alkalizing	Alkalizing	Acidifying	Strongly Acidifying
Apple cider vinegar	Almond Pesto (page 232)	Bouillon powder (MSG)	Artificial sweeteners (P)
	Beet and Almond Dip (page 230)	Honey, processed	Candied fruit (P)
	Celtic sea salt, unrefined sea salt (no anti-caking agent)	Hydrolyzed vegetable protein (MSG)	Caramels, toffee
	Gingerroot	Soy sauce (MSG, G)	Chewing gum (P)
	Halo Dressing (page 224)	Tamari (MSG)	Cocoa, chocolate (P)
	Herbal medicines	Tomato sauce, organic (MSG)	Gravy (MSG)
	Rice malt syrup	Vanilla extract	Ketchup (MSG)
	Soy lecithin granules	Wheat-free soy sauce (MSG)	Mayonnaise (P)
	Spices (such as cinnamon, ginger and saffron)		Mustard
	Vanilla, whole bean		Potato chips
			Salt, table/processed
			Sugar, granulated
			Sugar, raw/brown
			Table syrup
			Tomato paste (MSG)
			Vinegar, all but ACV

Protein: Legumes, Dairy, Seafood, Poultry, and Red Meat

Strongly Alkalizing	Alkalizing	Acidifying	Strongly Acidifying
	Egg yolk	Anchovies	Bacon
		Beans, cannellini (white kidney)	Beef
		Beans, fava	Cheese
		Beans, kidney	Custard
		Beans, navy	Deli meats, processed, seasoned (MSG)
		Chicken (skinless)	Fish, fried, pickled, smoked, salted
		Chickpeas	Herring Ω
		Egg whites	Ice cream
		Egg, whole, cooked	Kefir (fermented milk)
		Lamb	Lobster
		Lentils	Mackerel Ω
		Oysters	Meat pies (MSG)
		Sardines Ω	Pork (including ham)
		Soy milk, plain, organic (G)	Salmon, fresh Ω
		Soybeans (cooked)	Salmon, smoked Ω
		Trout, fresh Ω	Sausages (MSG)
		Tuna, fresh or canned Ω	Yogurt, sweetened
		Veal	
		White fish, fresh (see page 85 for low-mercury fish list) Ω	

Chapter 5

Balancing Your Diet

● ●

Take time to experiment with other foods that are low in dietary AGEs and rich in antioxidant nutrients and anthocyanins. Variety is not only the spice of life, it can also help you to look younger for longer. Eating a wide variety of healthy foods is part of the 28-day program for younger skin.

> Variety is not only the spice of life, it can also help you to look younger for longer.

Grains

Grains supply dietary fiber, which is essential for good bowel health and beautiful, blemish-free skin. Suitable flours and grains include spelt, rye, barley, quinoa, oats, and oat bran. Favor whole grains that have a low to medium GI rating. Basmati rice and sushi rice are okay because they have a medium to low GI, but many other white rice varieties have high glycemic index ratings. Avoid white bread, wheat flours, Turkish flatbread, and puffed amaranth because the glycemic index is incredibly high.

Spelt

Spelt is similar to wheat, but it is easier to digest because of its lower gluten content — so you are less likely to bloat after eating it (which can mean a flatter stomach). Spelt flour is a popular wheat flour alternative, especially for those intolerant to wheat. It bakes beautifully when used in cooking (almost rising as much as wheat) and it tastes remarkably similar to wheat.

FAQ

Q. I may have gluten intolerance. Is the diet suitable for me?

A. The 28-day program is a wheat-free diet, but it's not gluten-free. If you are sensitive to gluten, you will need to avoid wheat, oats, rye, barley, spelt, regular soy milk, and other products containing gluten. Substitute with rice, buckwheat, chickpeas or beans, flax seeds, lentils, quinoa, malt-free soy milk (or almond milk), and gluten-free pasta. If you suspect you are gluten intolerant, speak with your doctor about testing for celiac disease.

Did You Know?

No Added Yeast

Spelt sourdough bread uses the traditional, ambient yeast method of bread-making, so it is naturally lower in phytic acid. It also has a low GI — good news for keeping blood sugar levels steady, so there is less risk of AGE formation. If you cannot find spelt sourdough bread or spelt tortillas or wraps in your local area, you can bake your own flatbread — it's easy (see Spelt Flatbread, page 214). If you are gluten intolerant, stick with gluten-free alternatives, but first check if they're healthy, low GI, and free of artificial additives.

Oats

There's no need to buy expensive oats; just your regular rolled oats (which are super cheap) will do. I recommend soaking them overnight to make the nutrients more available and the cooking time quicker.

Rolled or traditional oats make a fantastic low-AGE breakfast. Oats are a cereal grain sometimes containing small amounts of gluten from cross-contamination. They are rolled flat, and this is how you want to buy them — not the ones that have been processed into instant oats. Extra processing gives them a higher GI, so they can spike blood sugar levels, which is bad news for the skin.

There's no need to buy expensive oats; just your regular rolled oats (which are super cheap) will do. I recommend soaking them overnight to make the nutrients more available and the cooking time quicker. To make a delicious non-toasted raw muesli recipe for younger-looking skin, try Omega Muesli (page 166). If you are allergic to gluten or oats, try Quinoa Porridge (page 168). Whenever consuming grains, add a dash of ground cinnamon to keep your blood sugar levels from spiking too much.

FAQ

Q. What if I have a negative reaction to a new food?

A. You could have an allergy, so take note if a food makes you feel unwell or itchy. You may need to vary the menu so that you are eating different foods each week, or introduce one new food every 3 days if you are not used to new products, such as flax seeds or pomegranate. If you experience symptoms after introducing a range of new products at once (for example, if you use a new skin cream and consume flaxseed oil and spelt bread), suspect an allergy or intolerance. In this case, go back to the "one new food/product every 3 days" rule — that is, introduce only one new food or product every 3 days, thus giving you time to see if you have an adverse reaction before introducing another new food or product. This will help you find what's right for you.

Protein Foods

Here are some guidelines for choosing quality protein foods, such as red meats (beef, pork, lamb), poultry (chicken, turkey), seafood (fish, shrimp), eggs, and soy products.

- Protein from animal sources should be free range and organic when possible.
- Avoid red meat for 28 days.
- If you like eating meat, favor skinless chicken and turkey.
- Skinless chicken or turkey can be eaten 1 or 2 times weekly, and fish/seafood 1 to 3 times weekly. On the other days, eat vegetarian options, such as soups.
- Remove chicken and turkey skin and cut off fatty pieces (the skin is incredibly rich in AGEs).

Thai cooking, where vegetables are stir-fried briefly, should contain only low to medium AGEs, and other vegetarian options are usually lowest in AGEs (as long as they are cheese-free).

- Buy only the freshest cuts of meat, free of preservatives and low in fat.
- If you are vegetarian, favor eggs, tofu, beans, and other legumes.
- Avoid vegetarian and vegan patties, plus meatless sausages; they can contain artificial additives and/or require frying.
- If you are vegan, make sure you eat legumes with a grain twice daily so you are consuming enough protein for healthy skin. For example, pair kidney beans, green beans, or raw tofu with rice or spelt pasta (plus veggies, of course).
- Avoid eating raw egg whites; they can cause what is known as egg white injury, a biotin deficiency that causes skin rashes and other skin problems.

FAQ

Q. What can I eat when I'm out at restaurants and cafés?

A. Sushi and Thai food are good choices. Thai cooking, where vegetables are stir-fried briefly, should contain only low to medium AGEs, and other vegetarian options are usually lowest in AGEs (as long as they are cheese-free). Avoid deep-fried foods, beef, and pork. Avoid curries that have been cooking for hours (vegetarian may be okay). Other options include:

- Casseroles
- Dal or other lentil dishes (no cream or cheese)
- Fish with steamed vegetables
- Rice (not fried rice)
- Salads
- Seafood marinara (tomato-based, no cream)
- Soups (no dairy, cream, or cheese)
- Stews
- Sushi, raw
- Tagines
- Thai stir-fried vegetables
- Vegetable curries (no dairy or cream)

Seafood

Studies show that eating 2 to 3 servings of fish each week is beneficial for elevating mood and increasing the health of the brain, skin, and heart. These benefits mainly come from the omega-3 fatty acids, EPA and DHA, found in seafood, particularly in oily fish. Good sources of these nutrients are trout, salmon, sardines, and herring (as well as fish oil supplements). Other minor sources of EPA and DHA are low-fat seafood, such as carp, pike, haddock, oysters, clams, scallops, and squid.

Choose seafood that is low in mercury. This heavy metal can be harmful to unborn babies and young children. It can also affect mental function and cause skin rashes. The general rule is: the higher up the food chain and the bigger the fish, the more mercury it could contain.

There are plenty of low-mercury choices, such as those listed under Good Seafood Choices, below. If in doubt, ask your local fishmonger.

> The higher up the food chain and the bigger the fish, the more mercury it could contain.

Good Seafood Choices

- Bream
- Catfish
- Dory (small fillets)
- Flounder
- Hake
- Herring
- Lobster
- Oysters
- Salmon
- Sardines
- Shrimp
- Trout and rainbow trout
- Tuna (a quality canned tuna in water/brine*)

* You can make a healthy snack with 3 ounces (90 g) of canned tuna twice weekly; canned tuna is sourced from smaller-sized tuna.

Fish to Avoid

The following fish contain high levels of mercury and should be avoided as often as possible:
- Cod (large fillets)
- King mackerel
- Marlin
- Perch (orange roughy)
- Snapper (larger fillets)
- Swordfish
- Tuna (larger fillets, albacore, southern bluefin)

Health authorities recommend that if you eat a serving of mercury-rich fish, you should then avoid eating all seafood for at least 2 weeks afterward to allow time for your mercury levels to reduce.

Legumes

Legumes are rich in magnesium and potassium and supply dietary fiber, protein, and slow-release carbohydrate for energy. Canned legumes, such as brown lentils, chickpeas, and mixed beans, are a convenient option, but I recommend cooking them fresh because the canned varieties may contain bisphenol A (BPA) — a substance used to coat the cans. The Food Standards Agency in the United Kingdom says that BPA is known to have weak estrogenic effects and could disrupt hormone systems. Dried legumes that are home-cooked are the best and most nutritious choice.

Cooking Guide for Legumes

Step 1: Rinsing

Rinse the legumes and pick out any discolored or shriveled specimens.

Step 2: Soaking

Soak the dried legumes to reduce phytic acid, promote even cooking, and reduce simmering time. Bring a large saucepan of water to boil and add the legumes; boil for 2 minutes. Remove from heat, cover, and soak overnight. Discard the soaking water; it contains the indigestible sugars that promote gas.

Step 3: Cooking

After soaking the legumes (if required), in a medium-sized saucepan, combine 4 cups (1 L) of water for every 1 cup (250 mL) of legumes. Cover with a lid and bring to a boil. Reduce to a simmer and check often. Avoid stirring the beans while cooking. Do not add salt; it can toughen the legumes if added too early.

Lentils are quick to cook, but for all other beans, check their progress after 45 minutes — if the legumes are cooked, they should be soft enough to easily mash using the back of a fork. All cooking times are approximate and will vary depending on how long it has been since the legumes were harvested.

Legume Cooking Times

Legume	Approximate cooking time
Adzuki beans	45 minutes–1½ hours
Black-eyed peas/beans	1–2 hours
Cannellini (white kidney) beans	1 hour
Chickpeas	1½–2 hours (let cool in cooking water)
Kidney beans	1 hour+
Lentils	20–30 minutes
Lima beans	1–2 hours
Mung beans	45–60 minutes
Navy beans	1–2 hours
Pinto beans	1–2 hours
Split peas, dried	Up to 45 minutes

FAQ

Q. What types of dried legumes do not need soaking?

A. Dried lentils (red and brown/green), split peas (green and yellow), and black-eyed peas do not need to be soaked, but you can soak them if you suffer from poor digestion. Adzuki and mung beans need to be soaked for only 1 to 2 hours. However, make sure you rinse these beans and lentils thoroughly, changing the water two or three times until it runs clear.

Oils

For 28 days, minimize cooking with oils, which are a rich source of AGEs. However, there are a couple of oils that are okay to use in moderation or raw in salads. Extra virgin olive oil that is cold-pressed may be used in salads and uncooked. The second option is rice bran oil that has been extra-cold-filtered — check the label when purchasing. Rice bran oil has one of the highest smoke points, making it okay for cooking at moderate temperatures if you must cook with oil.

Smoke Points of Common Cooking Oils

Cooking oil	Smoke point
Refined safflower oil	510°F (266°C)
Rice bran oil	490°F (254°C)
Ghee (Indian clarified butter)	485°F (252°C)
Refined/light olive oil	468°F (242°C)
Refined soybean oil	460°F (238°C)
Refined coconut oil	450°F (232°C)
Refined canola oil	400°F (204°C)
Extra virgin olive oil	375°F (190°C)
Extra virgin coconut oil	350°F (177°C)
Butter	250–300°F (121–149°C)
Virgin safflower oil	225°F (107°C)

Apple Cider Vinegar

Vinegar has been used for medicinal purposes and to flavor and preserve foods for more than 2,000 years. Today, unrefined apple cider vinegar is the therapeutic vinegar of choice because it is strongly alkalizing once digested (making it beneficial for the skin and the body's acid–alkaline balance). All other vinegars are strongly acidifying and are not recommended on a skin health program. (Other vinegars can be enjoyed in moderation as a part of a healthy diet after the 28-day program.)

According to research studies, apple cider vinegar has the added benefits of lowering blood sugar and delaying gastric emptying, so it can be beneficial for reducing glycation. Apple cider vinegar can be added to broths to help prevent AGE formation (see Anti-Aging Broth, page 184), or use apple cider vinegar to make salad dressings (see Halo Dressing, page 224; with frequent use, this salad dressing gives the skin a healthy glow).

Vinegar is strongly acidic before digestion, so it must be diluted with water or put into a dressing with other ingredients. Do not consume apple cider vinegar without diluting it first, and do not consume vinegar if you have gastric ulcers or sulfate sensitivity.

> Vinegar is strongly acidic before digestion, so it must be diluted with water or put into a dressing with other ingredients. Do not consume apple cider vinegar without diluting it first.

Rice Malt Syrup

Ideally, you should not consume added sweeteners, but for those of you who wish to use a sweetener, the best choice is rice malt syrup. There are two reasons: it is alkalizing (whereas all other sweeteners convert to acid in the body), and it has a very mild flavor, so it does not cause sugar cravings. It can be found in most health food shops and in some larger supermarkets.

Sea Salt

Commercial table salt usually contains an added anticaking agent with aluminum; most of the nutritious minerals have been removed; and it is acid-producing, so it can disrupt the body's acid–alkaline balance if used frequently. For these reasons it is best to avoid consuming commercial table salt.

If you would like to add salt to your meals, buy quality sea salt. The best salts are gray in color, indicating minimal processing and maximum mineral content. Quality sea salt may also be slightly damp or chunky, indicating an absence of anticaking agent. These alkaline salts are okay to use in moderation; however, do not add salt to your food if you have high blood pressure.

Non-Dairy Milks

Dairy products, especially animal milks (including cow, goat, and sheep milk), can contribute to excessively dry and prematurely aged skin and oily skin conditions, such as acne. Through my years of working with eczema sufferers and people with severe skin disorders, I have found that most skin problems can be improved by avoiding cow's milk and other dairy products, along with an increase in alkalizing foods in the diet.

According to an article published in the *Harvard Gazette*, dairy products are rich in animal sex hormones, and pregnant cows are commonly milked in Western countries, with their milk containing up to 33 times more estrogen than milk from a non-pregnant cow. A single cow provides almost 200,000 glasses of milk in her lifetime! The scientists from the Harvard School of Public Health went on to say that butter, milk, and cheese are implicated in higher rates of hormone-dependent cancers in humans, although more research is needed.

Organic Soy Milk

Unlike dairy milks, which are often rich in fats, lactose, and cholesterol, soy milk is low in saturated fat, is lactose-free, and can help to lower cholesterol and protect blood vessels from damage. Soy milk contains fewer sugars and calories than regular cow's milk, which has around 12 grams of sugar per cup (250 mL). This is because it's rich in lactose, a milk sugar. Compare this number to unsweetened soy milk, which has 1 to 4 grams per cup (250 mL).

Soy milk contains phytoestrogens, or plant estrogens, which are weaker than human or animal hormones. Research shows these phytoestrogens can be beneficial for people with low estrogen levels or those who are going through menopause. Phytoestrogens can promote calcium absorption in your body and this can reduce the risk of bone fractures and osteoporosis.

Like all processed food products, soy milk has its good and not-so-good points, and there are different qualities available. The best choice is soy milk containing organic whole soybeans because these are less processed and of the highest quality. Also choose one with added calcium, for bone health. Avoid soy milk that lists soy isolate as an ingredient; soy isolate was once considered a waste product and may contain aluminum. Furthermore, if you use soy milk made with whole soybeans, you're getting better (complete, or whole) protein, whereas soy milk made with isolate isn't a good protein source. If you have unusually high levels of estrogen in your body, soy milk may not be suitable for you; if you are concerned, your doctor can check your estrogen levels. Or just try delicious almond milk or rice milk (keep in mind that rice milk has a high GI, so you will need to add cinnamon to it).

FAQ

Q. Can people with gluten intolerance drink soy milk?

A. Yes, but you need to buy a specific type. The ingredient barley malt, which is added to most soy milks, contains gluten, so if you are gluten intolerant, look for malt-free soy milk or choose almond milk instead.

Almond Milk

Historically, almond milk was popular in medieval Europe and throughout the Middle East. Today it is gaining popularity once again as a high-protein alternative to regular cow's milk. Almonds supply vitamin E, magnesium, selenium, zinc, potassium, and calcium, plus a range of antioxidants, which can slow or inhibit AGE formation. Unlike cow's milk, which contains cholesterol, almond milk is cholesterol-free and has a cholesterol-lowering effect thanks to its flavonoid content.

Almond milk has a moisture-boosting effect on the skin, so if you have dry skin, this milk is for you. (However, if you have oily skin and breakouts occur after you change to almond milk, discontinue use. If you have acne or oily skin, organic soy milk would be your best choice.) Almond milk is available at health food shops and many supermarkets, but it's also super easy to make; the recipe is on page 172. Use the leftover almond meal as a body scrub to gently exfoliate your skin.

> Unlike cow's milk, which contains cholesterol, almond milk is cholesterol-free and has a cholesterol-lowering effect thanks to its flavonoid content.

Flax Seed Daily Intake

Adults with dry and aging skin can have 2 to 4 teaspoons (10 to 20 mL) of whole flax seeds daily, or 2 teaspoons (10 mL) of flaxseed oil, to boost skin moisture and promote smoother skin. Drink plenty of water when eating flax seeds because the fiber absorbs about five times the seeds' weight.

Flax Seeds

Flax seeds, also called linseeds, are small brown seeds best known for their rich content of anti-inflammatory omega-3 EFAs. The seeds are a source of phytochemicals, silica, mucilage, oleic acid, protein, vitamin E, and dietary fiber, for gastrointestinal and liver health. Flaxseed oil contains more than 50% omega-3 essential fatty acids and it's beneficial for dry skin conditions.

To demonstrate how essential fatty acids influence the skin, scientists gave two groups of women either flaxseed or borage oil — both rich sources of omega-3 and containing smaller amounts of omega-6 — and they gave a third group a placebo, which was olive oil. After 6 weeks of consuming only 1 teaspoon (15 mL) of either flaxseed oil or borage oil daily, skin water loss was decreased by about 10%, and by week 12, the flaxseed oil group showed further protection from water loss and the skin was significantly more hydrated. Although the olive oil (placebo) group showed no significant change in skin health, at 12 weeks, the flaxseed oil group had significantly less skin reddening, roughness, and scaling. Flax seeds can also accelerate wound healing and reduce inflammation and all-around skin sensitivity. Due to its moisture-boosting effect, flaxseed oil and flax seeds may not be suitable if you are prone to breakouts or have oily skin.

Storage Tips for Flaxseed Oil and Flax Seeds

Omega-3 EFAs are highly unstable and easily damaged by heat. Once flax seeds have been processed into oil or ground into a fine powder, they can go rancid within several weeks, especially if not stored correctly. For these reasons, do not buy pre-ground flax seeds or LSA (a mix containing ground flax seeds, sunflower seeds, and almonds). Instead, purchase whole flax seeds and grind them yourself at home just before using them.

Flaxseed oil must be refrigerated practically at all times. Flaxseed oil must not be heated or used for frying. Use it up within 4 or 5 weeks. However, whole flax seeds are easy to keep fresh; they are quite heat resistant, but store them in the refrigerator to increase shelf life.

Recommended recipes: they are great in smoothies (pages 173–174), or try Flaxseed Lemon Drink (page 175) and Omega Muesli (page 166).

> Flaxseed oil and flax seeds may not be suitable if you are prone to breakouts or have oily skin.

FAQ

Q. Can I eat omega-3-rich chia seeds?

A. Chia seeds have only recently become popular, and there is not a lot of scientific research on the health benefits of this tiny seed. However, we do know that they are a rich source of omega-3 (with more than 50% omega-3), so they can be a nutritious alternative to flax seeds.

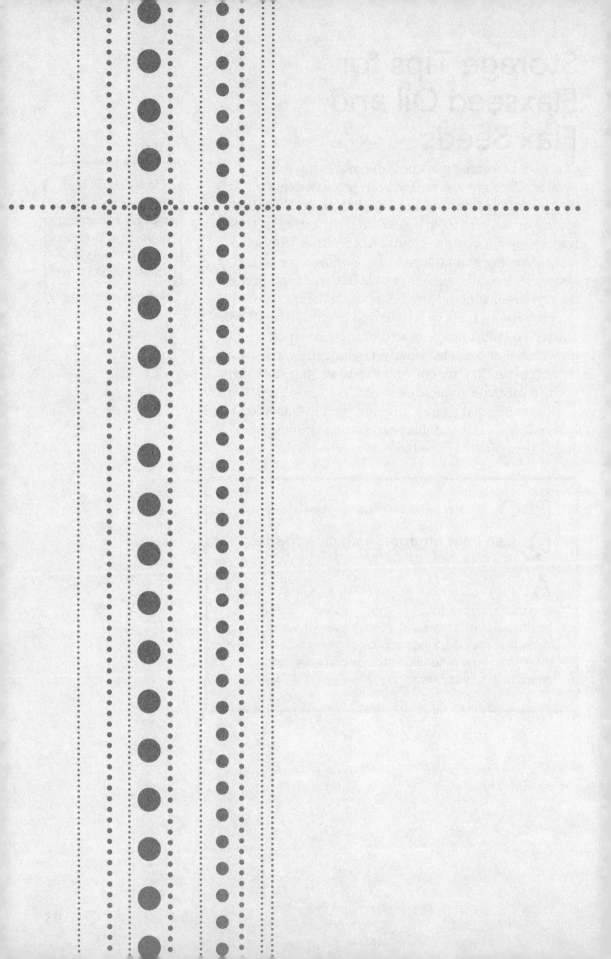

Chapter 6

Top 5 Anti-AGE Supplements

· ·

As you age, your skin becomes drier, nutrient levels decline, and wrinkle formation accelerates. Extra assistance through supplementation can help to slow some biochemical changes that occur with aging and to boost skin moisture so your skin appears more youthful. Here are the top five.

Health Note

Before taking supplements of any kind, seek advice from your doctor, especially if you are taking medical drugs or are pregnant or breastfeeding; the following supplements can have a detoxifying effect and may not be suitable for you. Some supplements, such as omega-3 and vitamin C, thin the blood. Avoid these supplements if you are on blood-thinning or heart medications or are preparing for surgery, laser treatments, injections, or childbirth. There are food alternatives for most supplements, so you can follow this program without supplements if needed.

---

1. Calcium

You may know that calcium is good for your bones and for calming the nervous system (thereby improving sleep), but what you may not realize is how important calcium is for your skin, especially the upper layer. Calcium promotes a healthy acid mantle, which protects your skin from microbe invasion and infections. The epidermis layer of the skin must also respond to weather extremes, and calcium helps to maintain the right amount of moisturizing lipids by triggering their production in low humidity or when required. These lipids are water resistant, trapping water in the skin so it does not dry out.

Low calcium levels in the epidermis hamper the skin's natural exfoliating process. This causes dead skin cells to build up, leading to greater premature aging and skin that appears dry and dull.

The Research...

- In healthy skin, high concentrations of calcium and magnesium are present in the upper epidermis.
- If the moisture level in the air drops, calcium triggers the skin to increase the production of lipids, and the epidermis thickens in order to trap moisture in your skin.
- Intake of calcium, retinol, and the collagen-promoting nutrients vitamin C, magnesium, iron, and zinc appear to be protective against UV-induced skin aging.

The calcium paradox is that dairy products, which are rich in calcium, can contribute to skin problems, such as acne, eczema, and cellulite (possibly due to the presence of animal hormones and high AGEs and the absence of the right supporting nutrients), but calcium in supplement form has a youth-promoting effect on aging skin. Calcium, when taken with a healthy diet and with magnesium, vitamin D, and collagen-supporting nutrients zinc, manganese, and copper, helps to tighten up connective tissue and reduces the appearance of cellulite and sagging skin within 28 days.

Dosage Information

Dosage for adults: 1000 to 1200 mg of calcium daily in divided doses, taken in between meals so it does not interfere with the absorption of other minerals. If you are postmenopausal, pregnant, breastfeeding, or have poor bone density, take 1200 mg daily. Ideally, choose a calcium supplement that contains a combination of calcium citrate (avoid calcium carbonate), vitamin D, magnesium, zinc, manganese, and copper.

Caution

Calcium supplementation can interfere with drug absorption. Speak with your doctor before taking calcium if you are on medication or are unwell. Do not take antacids containing aluminum while taking calcium.

FAQ

Q. Do I need to supplement my diet with liquid chlorophyll?

A. Chlorophyll is the green pigment found in plants. It absorbs sunlight and converts it to plant energy. Chlorophyll is highly alkalizing; it contains potassium and iron; and it is rich in magnesium, which is needed for cardiovascular and skin health. Chlorophyll increases oxygen-carrying capacity in the blood, which can give you more energy and stamina, and it has a blood-thinning effect, which gives the skin a healthy glow. It promotes friendly bacteria in the bowel, so it can reduce harmful bowel microbes; it promotes healthy digestion; and chlorophyll prevents bad breath and body odor.

If you don't think you are getting enough greens in your diet, consider taking a liquid chlorophyll supplement for skin health (available at health food shops and online). Just mix a teaspoon or two (5 or 10 mL) in a glass of water. Please note that using liquid chlorophyll is optional.

2. Vitamin C

The body is truly remarkable and resourceful. It makes many of its own vitamins in the gastrointestinal tract and it stores minerals in the liver and bones; however, the body does not store or manufacture vitamin C, so it must be consumed in your diet every day. Vitamin C (also known as ascorbic acid) aids in the absorption of iron and copper, boosts the formation of collagen in the skin, guards against infections, and is required for liver detoxification. Vitamin C also inhibits glycation and AGE formation, so it is an important anti-aging nutrient.

> Allergy sufferers must avoid developing vitamin C deficiency because it can result in histamine toxicity, and allergic reactions may increase in severity.

Vitamin C is a natural antihistamine that destroys the imidazole ring of the histamine molecule. For this reason, allergy sufferers must avoid developing vitamin C deficiency because it can result in histamine toxicity, and allergic reactions may increase in severity. You need to consume at least 45 mg of vitamin C every day to avoid developing a deficiency, but higher amounts are needed to reduce the severity of allergies, boost collagen production in the skin, and enjoy optimal health. See page 112 for vitamin C deficiency symptoms.

Dosage Information

Dosage for adults: consume between 50 and 200 mg of vitamin C daily from foods — the menus in this book will help you do this. Because ascorbic acid (the general form of vitamin C) is acidic, when buying a supplement, look for buffered vitamin C, which has an added alkaline mineral, such as magnesium ascorbate, potassium ascorbate, sodium ascorbate, or calcium ascorbate.

Caution

Vitamin C thins the blood. Do not take vitamin C supplements if you have hemochromatosis or if you have been prescribed aspirin, anticoagulants, or antidepressants. See Health Note on page 95.

Food Sources of Vitamin C

Food sources	Vitamin C content in mg per 3½ oz (100 g) (unless specified)
Guava	245 mg
Red bell pepper	170 mg
Brussels sprouts	110 mg
Broccoli	105 mg
Green bell pepper	90 mg
Cauliflower	70 mg
Papaya	60 mg
Strawberries (1 cup/250 mL)	55 mg
Lemon (1 medium)	50 mg
Sweet potato	30 mg
White potato	30 mg

3. Chromium

The mineral chromium is required in micro amounts for normal growth and general health, and for the breakdown of proteins, carbohydrates, and fats. It is the active ingredient in glucose tolerance factor (a compound that helps in blood sugar regulation) and it enhances the action of the hormone insulin, which helps your body control glucose in the blood. Chromium's action of helping the body to correctly process glucose (blood sugar) for energy use reduces the risk of advanced glycation end products and protects collagen from irreparable damage. It can also dampen sugar cravings. Deficiency symptoms are listed on page 108.

Although statistics on chromium deficiency are limited, data from research suggest that only 0.4% to 2.5% of chromium is absorbed from foods. Vitamin C and vitamin B_3 (niacin) enhance the absorption of chromium, as does protein, so take a chromium supplement with a protein-rich meal. Chromium picolinate is easier for the body to absorb than other types of chromium, and a chromium supplement should also contain vitamins B_3, B_6, B_{12}, vitamin C, vitamin D_3, folic acid, magnesium, and zinc.

> Chromium is the active ingredient in glucose tolerance factor (a compound that helps in blood sugar regulation) and it enhances the action of the hormone insulin, which helps your body control glucose in the blood.

Dosage Information

Dosage for adults: Between 45 and 60 mcg (µg) elemental chromium daily from foods and supplement. It is ideal to have a chromium supplement in divided doses with each main meal. Note that "mcg" is also written as "µg."

Caution

If you are taking medical drugs, consult with a nutritionist or doctor before taking chromium. If you have insulin-dependent diabetes, seek advice from your doctor before supplementing with chromium because it alters blood sugar levels (insulin would need to be reduced if you were taking chromium, but do this only with your doctor's supervision).

Food Sources of Chromium

Food source	Chromium content (in mcg)
Romaine lettuce (2 cups/500 mL)	16
Onion, raw (½ cup/125 mL)	12
Turkey (3½ oz/100 g)	10
Peas, cooked (1 cup/250 mL)	6
Garlic powder (1 tsp/5 mL)	3
Potato, mashed (1 cup/250 mL)	3
Bread, whole-grain (2 slices)	2
Banana (1 medium)	1
Green beans (½ cup/125 mL)	1

4. Essential Fatty Acids

EPA and DHA calm skin inflammation, reduce skin sensitivity, and enhance the immune system (they're great for the heart, too).

Essential fatty acids (EFAs) are vital for healthy skin and are classified as "essential" because your body cannot manufacture them and they must be obtained from your diet. The two main groups of essential fatty acids are omega-3 and omega-6. Omega-6 is present in vegetable oils, margarine, nuts, and seeds and is usually overconsumed in the Western diet (which can lead to oily skin and blemishes if you are prone to these conditions).

Rich sources of omega-3 are flax seeds, chia seeds, fresh walnuts, and fish, especially trout, salmon, and sardines. Omega-3 works to create younger skin in a number of ways. It converts to potent anti-inflammatory substances called EPA (eicosapentaenoic acid) and DHA (docosahexaenoic acid), which are omega-3 in its more potent form. EPA and DHA calm skin inflammation, reduce skin sensitivity, and enhance the immune system (they're great for the heart, too).

Balancing the Fats in Your Diet

Both omega-6 and omega-3 make a noticeable difference to oil production and the moisture content of the skin, but you should consume them in a 1:1 ratio (in typical Western diets, the ratio is more like 20:1). To amend the ratios of these fats in your diet, eat fewer processed vegetable oils (and fewer fatty meats), ditch margarine, and add fish, seafood, and/or flax seeds to your diet. If you are vegetarian or vegan, favor fresh walnuts, flax seeds, or chia seeds. Dark leafy greens also contain small amounts of omega-3.

Dosage Information

To avoid deficiency, your EPA/DHA dosage should be at least 600 mg daily. Adults who want to treat very dry skin, wrinkles, and premature aging can take up to 2000 mg EPA/DHA daily in divided doses (approximately 6 grams of omega-3 depending on the brand, but lower doses may also be effective). On the days you eat fresh fish or seafood, you can skip taking an omega-3 supplement. If you do not want to take fish oil supplements or eat fish, just add flax seeds and flaxseed oil to your diet (see page 92).

> On the days you eat fresh fish or seafood, you can skip taking an omega-3 supplement.

Caution

Omega-3 has many benefits, but supplements are not suitable for everyone. Do not take flaxseed oil or high-dose omega-3 oils if you have acne or are prone to breakouts; doing so may increase skin oiliness. Read the Health Note on page 95 to see if this supplement is right for you.

Food Sources of Omega-3

Food (standard servings)	Omega-3 content* (in mg)
Salmon (4 oz/114 g)	2000
Flax seeds (1 tbsp/15 mL)	1750
Eggs, omega-3 fortified (2 eggs)	1114
Scallops (4 oz/114 g)	1100
Halibut, baked (4 oz/114 g)	620

Food Sources of EPA and DHA

Note: These are active/therapeutic compounds with omega-3.

Food (3½ oz/100 g unless specified)	EPA/DHA content (in mg)
Herring	1710–1810*
Atlantic salmon	1090–1830*
Sardines	980–1700*
Flaxseed oil (1 tbsp/15 mL)	850
Rainbow trout	840–980*
Mackerel	340–1570*
Tuna, canned in water, drained	260–730*
Tuna, fresh	240–1280*
Flax seeds, ground or whole (1 tbsp/15 mL)	220

* The EPA and DHA content varies depending on whether the skin has been left on or removed: fish with skin on is higher in fat, so it is a richer source of omega-3 fatty acids, EPA, and DHA.

5. Carotenoids

> Carotenoids, such as beta-carotene and cryptoxanthin, are potent AGE inhibitors and should be consumed daily.

Research shows that eating foods rich in cryptoxanthin, a carotenoid that supplies vitamin A, significantly boosts skin hydration. Carotenoids, such as beta-carotene and cryptoxanthin, are potent AGE inhibitors and should be consumed daily — but preferably not in supplement form because they work best when packaged in fresh fruits and vegetables.

Cryptoxanthin-rich foods are papaya, pumpkin, paprika, persimmons, bell peppers, and peaches. Carrots, beets, and sweet potatoes are some examples of beta-carotene-rich foods.

Dosage Information

Have at least 1 serving of carotenoid-rich fruit or vegetables daily — at least half a cup (125 mL). Recipes include Peach, Thyme and Chile Marinade (page 216), Papaya Cups with Lime and Guava (page 226), Mediterranean Seafood Soup (page 190), Spiced Sweet Potato Soup (page 187), and Sweet Potato Salad (page 195).

Nutrients for Collagen Production

If you were to build a house, you would ideally use a supply of strong, weather-resistant materials, such as timber, concrete, nails, bricks, and so on. Then as the years passed by, you would repair any breakages, give it a new coat of paint, and — if the roof leaked — you would maybe replace a few tiles and fix the guttering. It's a similar story with your skin: you need to supply the right building materials from your diet so that your body can make healthy skin, and then you need a constant supply of the right nutrients for the maintenance, repair, and renewing of skin cells and collagen.

Recall that collagen is like the glue that holds your skin firmly in place and gives it resilience. But collagen does not magically appear or stay the same once it's formed. More than one-third of collagen is made up of the amino acid

> You need to supply the right building materials from your diet so that your body can make healthy skin, and then you need a constant supply of the right nutrients for the maintenance, repair, and renewing of skin cells and collagen.

glycine, another third is proline, and the rest consists of lysine and other amino acids, supplied by protein-containing foods, such as fish, eggs, meats, beans, nuts, and seeds. Lysine and proline need co-factors vitamin C, iron, and manganese to form strong collagen in the skin, and zinc is vital for collagen formation.

If your diet lacked even just one of the right collagen-building nutrients, it would be like holidaying in a house made of straw or bamboo — it might look like a Balinese resort online, but in reality it's a building that leaks whenever it rains and there is never a repairman when you need one. Your diet might consist of the most decadent foods (see the Prisoner Study, below), but without the right nutrients to aid the structural formation of collagen, the skin, tendons, and blood vessels become fragile, your skin can become oversensitive to its environment (the weather, skin products, and pollen, to name a few), and skin aging is accelerated.

Prisoner Study

In 1969, six prisoners were involved in a scientific diet experiment that involved eating pancakes, bacon, cooked egg whites, noodles, and butterscotch pudding with marshmallows and meringue. They also ate chocolate, candy, muffins, seafood, chicken casseroles, and gingerbread cookies, and they drank strawberry-flavored soft drink (a diet similar to what some children and Western families eat today). However, vitamin C was missing from the diet. To ensure it was the only deficiency the prisoners experienced (going without vitamin C could have caused a few malnutrition problems), they were given a vitamin and mineral supplement that supplied everything except for vitamin C.

After 3 weeks of being on this decadent diet, the scientists reported the prisoners' gums started to swell and bleed, and their skin developed small bumps, which worsened over time. Several men developed infections, including sore throat, ear infection, and fevers. Two of the inmates escaped at this point. The rest of the prisoners continued with the diet until their skin literally began to fall apart. On Day 36 of the diet, one prisoner had to have two teeth removed, and the prisoners complained of fatigue and muscle cramps. On the 52nd day, mild hemorrhaging of the skin and follicles occurred, blood spotting began in the eyes, and skin bumpiness increased as collagen could no longer form properly without vitamin C. The study, published in the *American Journal of Clinical Nutrition*, was halted at this point. (*Note:* This study was conducted in the days before the ethical implications of conducting experiments on prisoners were a consideration.)

FAQ

Q. How many supplements do I need to take for younger skin?

A. First, read the Health Note on page 95 to check if supplementation is right for you. If you are okay to take supplements, you can take the following:

1. Calcium supplement with added vitamin D (daily, taken before breakfast and dinner)
2. Chromium, with added vitamins C, B_3, and B_6, plus magnesium, manganese, and zinc (daily, taken with breakfast and lunch)
3. If you are a woman or a vegetarian or vegan, take an herbal iron supplement daily to boost collagen production in the skin; see iron information on page 106

Your diet should supply the other nutrients for healthy skin, and the menus and shopping list in Part 2 will make this easy for you.

The only reasons to take an additional supplement would be if you have deficiency symptoms or if you have been prescribed a supplement for medical reasons. Complete the Nutrient Deficiency Questionnaire (at 108) to see if you need to take additional supplements (or have a health checkup).

Nutrients for Collagen Formation

Here is a list of the nutrients your body absolutely needs to build strong and healthy collagen. They can all be obtained through your diet.

Nutrient for collagen formation + daily intake	Food sources (nutrient content per 3½ oz/100 g unless otherwise specified)	
Protein (supplies amino acids, such as glycine, proline, and lysine) AI: 1 g of protein per 2 lbs (1 kg) of body weight daily (more for athletes) RDA: 56 g for men; 46 g for women (71 g if pregnant or breastfeeding)	5 oz (150 g) cooked chicken (42 g) 5 oz (150 g) cooked fish (36 g) Canned tuna or salmon (24 g) 1 cup (250 mL) cooked legumes (16 g) 6 jumbo shrimp (14 g) 1 large egg (6 g)	
Glycine (one-third of collagen is made up of this amino acid; protein foods are rich in glycine) Recommended intake: 2–5 g	Anti-Aging Broth (page 184) (1904 mg) ⅓ oz (10 g) unsweetened gelatin powder (1904 mg) Soybeans, raw (1880 mg) Turkey or chicken, with skin (1395 mg) Split peas (1092 mg) Crab (1089 mg) Tuna, raw (1056 mg) Buckwheat (1031 mg) Salmon, raw (1022 mg) Red lentils (1014 mg) Rainbow trout (1002 mg) ⅔ oz (20 g) flax seeds (250 mg)	
Iron RDA: 8 mg for men; 18 mg for women (27 mg if pregnant)	Green pumpkin seeds (10 mg) Mussels (8 mg) Soy milk (7–9 mg) Tempeh (7 mg) Oysters (6 mg) 1 cup (250 mL) cooked lentils (4 mg) Scallops (3 mg) Tofu (3 mg) Whole-grain bread (3 mg) Chicken (1 mg) 1 tbsp (15 ml) tahini (1 mg)	
Zinc AI: 8 mg RDA: 11 mg for men; 8 mg for women (11 to 12 mg if pregnant or breastfeeding) Recommended intake: 14–20 mg	Oysters (45 mg) Whole-grain bread (8 mg) Sardines, canned (5 mg) Brazil nuts (4 mg) Crab (4 mg) Eggs, poached (4 mg)	Almonds (3 mg) Apricots, dried (3 mg) Chicken (2 mg) Rolled oats (2 mg) Lentils (1 mg) Salmon (1 mg)

Nutrient for collagen formation + daily intake	Food sources (nutrient content per 3½ oz/100 g unless otherwise specified)
Manganese AI: 2 mg RDA: 2.3 mg for men; 1.8 mg for women (2.0 mg if pregnant; 2.6 mg if breastfeeding)	Spelt (1.9 mg) 1 cup (250 mL) cooked chickpeas (1.7 mg) Oat bran muffin (1.5 mg) 1 cup (250 mL) cooked oatmeal (1.3 mg) ½ cup (125 mL) brown rice (1.1 mg) 1 cup (250 mL) cooked lima beans (1.1 mg) 1 cup (250 mL) green tea (1.0 mg) 1 cup (250 mL) mashed cooked sweet potato (0.9 mg) 1 handful almonds (0.7 mg) 1 cup (250 mL) black tea (0.5 mg)
Silicon (silica) Recommended intake: 10–25 mg	Beans, green or French (8.7 mg) Dates, dried (16 mg) (3 dates = 7 mg) Oat bran (23 mg) (2 tbsp/30 mL bran = 3 mg) Oat cereals/granola (12 mg) Oats, porridge (11 mg) Red lentils (4 mg) Spinach, fresh, boiled (5 mg) Wheat bran cereal (11 mg) Whole-grain bread (5 mg)
Vitamin C AI: 45 mg RDA: 90 mg for men; 75 mg for women (85 mg if pregnant; 120 mg if breastfeeding) Recommended intake: 50–200 mg	See page 98
Copper AI: 1.7 mg Recommended intake: 2–3 mg	Oysters (7.6 mg) Mushrooms (0.6 mg) Crab (4.8 mg) Spinach (0.3 mg) Brazil nuts (1.1 mg) Sweet potato (0.2 mg) Whole-grain bread (0.8 mg) Salmon (0.1 mg) Shrimp (0.7 mg)

AI = adequate intake for adults to avoid deficiency
RDA = recommended dietary allowance as per U.S. Department of Agriculture (USDA) guidelines
Recommended intake = my recommended daily intake for younger skin

Nutrient Deficiency Questionnaire

What is your body trying to tell you? We are often taught to accept ourselves the way we are, but what if your skin problems are trying to tell you something important about your health? Nutritional deficiencies accelerate skin aging and cause a range of unpleasant symptoms that can worsen over time and lead to serious health complications if left untreated. Check if you have signs of nutritional deficiencies by circling any signs and symptoms you have in the following questionnaire. Please note that the following symptoms can be caused by other factors and this questionnaire does not take the place of medical advice. An asterisk (*) denotes a symptom that you may need to discuss with your doctor in order to rule out other factors.

Nutrient	Signs and Symptoms of Deficiency
Calcium	Cellulite and/or poor skin tone Cramps or aches* Dry skin Excessive irritability or nerves Insomnia* Lethargy Muscle twitching* Numbness; tingling fingers*, arms, and/or legs* Poor appetite* Rickets, poor bone health,* osteoporosis* Stiff sore neck, ribcage pain, backache*
Chromium	Acne/pimples* ADD/ADHD* Anxiety attacks* Cravings for sweets, carbs, or alcohol Depression* Excessive thirst* Fatigue in between meals High blood sugar (pre-diabetes, type 2 diabetes)* Hypoglycemia/low blood sugar Irritability or dizziness after 2 to 6 hours without food* Need for frequent meals Poor concentration* Premature aging
Copper	Age spots Impaired growth* Liver cancer* Loss of pigmentation Muscle disease* Neurological symptoms* Sagging skin

Essential Fatty Acids (Omega-3 and/or Omega-6)	Arthritis* Bumps on the backs of upper arms Depression* Dry skin Dry, brittle hair or dandruff Frequent infections Hyperactivity, ADD/ADHD* Infertility* Learning difficulties Poor vision Poor wound healing* Skin rashes Weakness
Folate (Vitamin B$_9$)	Anemia* Cracked lips and corners of mouth Depression* Diarrhea* Forgetfulness or sluggishness Gastrointestinal disorders* Inflamed tongue Insomnia* Irritability or hostility* Pallor/pale complexion* Shortness of breath*
Iodine	Constipation* Depression* Dry skin and hair Infertility* Intolerance to cold weather Low sex drive* Miscarriages* Puffiness under eyes Slow metabolism* Swollen neck (goiter)* Unexplained weight gain*
Iron	Anemia* Constipation* Cravings for ice, clay, or starch Dizziness* Heart palpitations* Labored breathing* Pale eyelid rims (should be pink) Pale palm creases Pallor or grayish skin* Ridges lengthwise in nails Sore tongue Split fingernails that won't heal Spoon-shaped nails

continued...

Magnesium	Anxiety or irritability Clicking joints Convulsions* Cravings for alcohol or sugar Insomnia* Irregular heartbeat* Muscle cramps or pain* Muscle twitching or weakness* PMS Soft or brittle nails Tender calf muscles
Manganese	Abnormal blood sugar levels Bone malformations* Convulsions* Elevated blood calcium (in test results) Growing pains during childhood Impaired growth* Iron-deficiency anemia* Muscle twitching Poor balance Skin rash Weakness or dizziness*
Molybdenum	Headaches* Night blindness* Rapid breathing* Rapid heart rate* Sensitivity to chemicals Sensitivity to sulfates and sulfur
Potassium	Abdominal pain* Abnormal heartbeat* Bloating Constipation* Fatigue* Hypokalemia* Intestinal paralysis* Muscle weakness and cramps* Tetany (muscle spasms)
Selenium	Inability to cope with stress* Inflammation or damaged heart muscles* Liver cancer* Muscle weakness and wasting* Poor immunity
Silica	Bone abnormalities* Brittle fingernails Dry, brittle, or thin hair Joint problems* Premature aging

Vitamin A and Beta-Carotene	Acne Bumpy skin on backs of upper arms Dandruff Diarrhea* Dry eyes Frequent colds or infections Mouth ulcers Poor night vision Rough skin on heels Scaly and dry skin
Vitamin B_1 (Thiamine)	Burning feet Constipation* General weakness* Irritability Loss of appetite* Muscle atrophy* Nervous conditions* Pins and needles/numbness* Poor circulation* Rapid heartbeat*
Vitamin B_2 (Riboflavin)	Broken capillaries on face Dermatitis Increased sensitivity to light Loss of eyebrows/hair loss* Mouth sores Oily or dull hair Red, sore tongue Sore or gritty feeling in eyes Sore, dry, or cracked lips Split nails
Vitamin B_3 (Niacin)	Bleeding gums* Blood sugar problems Cracked corners of mouth Depression* Dermatitis Diarrhea* Low energy Muscular weakness* Pimples Red, rough skin
Vitamin B_6 (Pyridoxine)	Acne Anemia* Convulsions* Cracked skin at corners of mouth Dermatitis Frequent colds or flu Low blood sugar/hypoglycemia Mood changes/irritability Muscle weakness* Numbness or cramps in arms or legs* Smooth, painful tongue* *continued...*

continued...

Vitamin B$_7$ (Biotin)	Anxiety/inability to cope* Dandruff Depression* or moodiness Dermatitis or eczema Dry skin Grayish skin color or pallor* Localized numbness* Loss of appetite* Muscle pain* Premature graying of hair Red, scaly skin around eyes* Scaly lips
Vitamin B$_{12}$ (Cobalamin)	Anemia* Constipation* Dark, thin, or spoon-shaped nails Depression* Fatigue Nervousness or anxiety* Numb/tingling hands and feet* Pallor/pasty complexion Poor coordination Red, smooth tongue Shortness of breath*
Vitamin C (Ascorbic Acid)	Allergies* Anemia* Bumpy/rough skin or rash Cravings for sweets or fruit Depression* Dry skin Easy bruising or small purplish spots on skin* Fatigue Fluid retention or swelling of lower limbs* Frequent colds and flu Frequent nosebleeds* Hemorrhaging* Poor wound healing* Swollen or bleeding gums Tooth loss*
Vitamin D	Bone deformities* Eczema or psoriasis Fatigue Frequent backache* Joint pain or stiffness* Muscle twitching or spasms* Muscle weakness* Osteoporosis* Rickets/bowed legs*

Vitamin E (D-Alpha-Tocopherol) (deficiency is rare)	Abnormal eye movements* Anemia* Dry skin Frequent diarrhea with fat in stools* Gluten intolerance* Infertility* Loss of delicate sense of touch* Miscarriages* Poor balance/equilibrium* Premature aging* Restless legs* Skin inflammation*
Vitamin K (deficiency is rare)	Blood oozing from gums or nose* Easily fractured bones* Easy bruising Excessive bleeding from cuts (slow to clot)* Osteoporosis*
Zinc	Acne or oily skin Anorexia or poor appetite* Diarrhea* Frequent infections* or colds/flu Frizzy hair or hair loss Impotence* Infertility* Poor sense of taste or smell Poor wound healing* Ridges on fingernails Skin lesions* Split, brittle, or peeling fingernails Stretch marks White spots on fingernails White-coated tongue

Analyzing the Questionnaire

If you have three or more symptoms (in a category), you may have a deficiency that requires supplementation or further investigation. However, a single unpleasant symptom can be an early warning sign that you have a mineral deficiency requiring attention. For example, if you have a split fingernail that won't heal, you should investigate the cause — it could be something as simple as early iron deficiency caused by drinking tea during meals (because the tannins bind with iron from the meal, making it unavailable for absorption).

If you find you have many nutrient deficiencies, it could indicate any of the following: digestive problems, malabsorption, candidiasis/fungal infestation, malnutrition, poor diet, excess alcohol consumption, early disease states, or excess laxative use, to name a few.

Unpleasant symptoms are your body's way of saying, "Look after me and investigate further." If symptoms don't quickly improve with supplementation, speak with your doctor or health-care professional for a formal diagnosis.

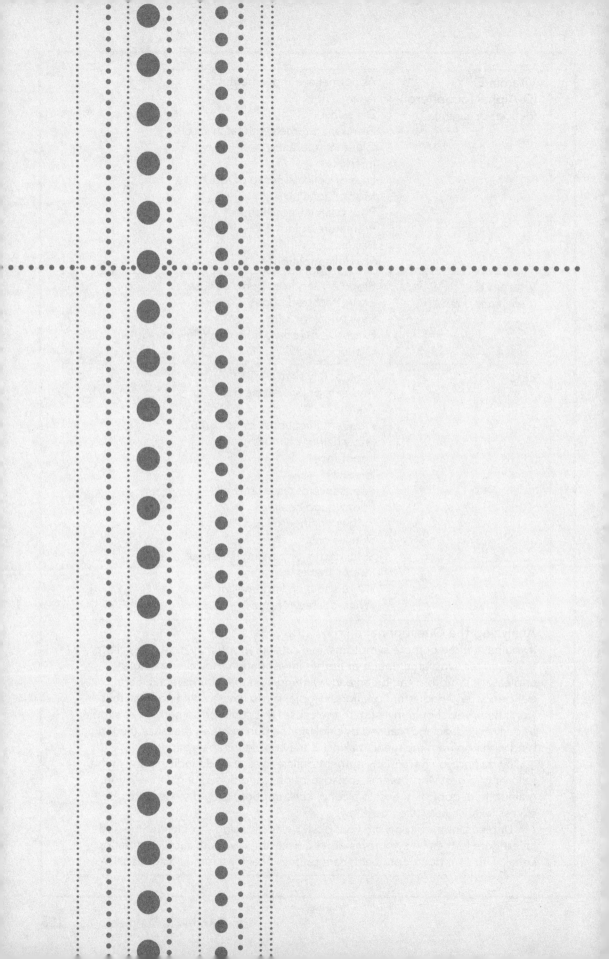

Chapter 7

Choosing Skin Beauty Products

• •

As a complement to the nutritional strategies outlined in this book, some skin beauty products can make your skin younger. By choosing beauty products that contain active ingredients, you can do more than moisturize your skin — you can create smoother skin, stimulate the production of new collagen, encourage faster cell renewal, and make your skin look younger! The right skin-care ingredients can also help to protect your skin from environmental damage and UV radiation. There are many, many skin-care ingredients that are great for moisturizing the skin (and I will cover these, too), but this chapter focuses on the top five active skin-care ingredients for creating younger skin. I have also included some guidelines for choosing and using makeup to your best advantage.

Beautifully applied makeup — that looks natural and highlights your features — can hide age spots and whatever else your diet and skin-care regimen cannot fix. I highly recommend investing in a makeup book and learning from a makeup expert. Free makeup consultations are often available from specialty makeup stores. Look for makeup books written specifically for your age group.

> The right skin-care ingredients can also help to protect your skin from environmental damage and UV radiation.

What to Look For

There are literally thousands of skin-care ingredients, so what do you look for when buying a product? When your skin is young, you might just pop a bit of shea butter moisturizer on your skin and you're set for the day. However, as you age, you may find that the basic products might moisturize your skin, but they don't reduce real signs of aging — namely wrinkles, sun spots, mottled pigmentation, and creases on your chest when you wake in the morning! Thankfully, scientists from around the globe who have an interest in skin care have determined the most active ingredients in skin care today.

FAQ

Q. Do I need to change my skin-care routine?

A. Your skin-care routine should suit your lifestyle, your skin type, and your budget. If you already like your skin-care routine and if you prefer to focus on your diet during the 28 days, that is fine. Just ensure your skin-care products aren't causing breakouts or drying out your skin. If you are under 30 years old and already have good skin, you might not need to change your skin-care routine, but if you have sun-damaged skin, a bit of extra assistance can help you look years younger. Later in this chapter there are examples of skin-care regimens for those who want to try something new.

Retinyl palmitate is one of the main antioxidants found naturally in the skin and it helps to guard against the damaging effects of free radicals and UV radiation. However, this natural antioxidant depletes every time your skin is exposed to sunlight.

1. Retinol

Retinol is a pure form of vitamin A that improves the texture and appearance of aging skin. Clinical trials consistently show that topically applied retinol stimulates the production of new collagen and glycosaminoglycans (GAGs), which hold water and have a plumping effect on the skin. Retinyl palmitate is one of the main antioxidants found naturally in the skin and it helps to guard against the damaging effects of free radicals and UV radiation. However, this natural antioxidant depletes every time your skin is exposed to sunlight, so it is vital to restore vitamin A levels within the skin each day, especially as you age. When shopping for face moisturizers or treatments, look for names such as retinol, retinyl palmitate, retinoic acid, adapalene, and tretinoin in the list of ingredients.

Benefits of retinol in skin care*	Guidelines
Stimulates production of procollagen and collagen Increases glycosaminoglycans (GAGs) Increases dermal matrix of skin Minimizes fine lines and wrinkles Repairs some sun-induced skin aging Improves functioning of skin cells Causes firmer skin (when added to cellulite products) Decreases skin roughness Increases protection from ulcer formation	Improvement within 28 days Best results in 24 weeks to 12 months (if using a low dose and working up to a stronger dose) Suitable for most skin types, but sensitive skin may need time to adjust — or begin on a low dose Do not apply over eczema, skin rashes, or broken skin Wear a hat and/or use sunscreen daily when using retinol products

* Topical 0.4% retinol lotion was applied on the skin of elderly patients 3 times weekly for 24 weeks to obtain results.

High-dose retinol can irritate the skin, so it is advisable to start on a low dose and acclimatize your skin, especially if you have sensitive skin. Some research shows that lower doses are just as effective as the higher prescription-only doses. Refer to online product review websites.

FAQ

Q. Do I begin a new skin-care routine at the same time as changing my diet?

A. Ideally, you want to keep the two separate so that you can see if a skin-care product is right for you. If you drastically change your diet and start using new skin-care products on the same day and your skin breaks out, it will be hard to tell if it is a reaction to the skin-care product or if you are sensitive to a particular food or if you are experiencing a typical detox symptom. It is recommended to start the new diet program at least a few days beforehand. You will probably need to take your time choosing the right skin-care products for your skin type (and budget!), and testing the products in the store or asking for samples can help. Also, you may have to wait for products to be in stock or be sent to you if ordering online; this can delay the beginning of your skin-care routine.

2. AHAs and BHA

Alpha-hydroxy acids (AHAs) and salicylic acid (beta-hydroxy acid, or BHA) speed up skin-cell renewal by helping to remove the substances that hold dead skin cells together and they have an exfoliating effect.

As you age, your skin-cell turnover rate decreases by 30% to 50%, which causes a buildup of dead skin cells. Alpha-hydroxy acids (AHAs) and salicylic acid (beta-hydroxy acid, or BHA) speed up skin-cell renewal by helping to remove the substances that hold dead skin cells together and they have an exfoliating effect — so your skin is left feeling smoother and softer. AHAs and BHA in skin care also improve the skin's texture by forcing the skin to renew itself more quickly than it normally would and without damaging the skin's protective barrier. They work by setting off a wound-healing response in the dermis layer of the skin, which triggers increased collagen production. The eventual result is a visible reduction in sun-damaged skin, fewer wrinkles, and a more even skin tone.

AHAs and BHA can help to reduce acne scars, but it won't happen overnight and long-term use is necessary. Salicylic acid (BHA) is added to pimple cream formulas because it reduces swelling and speeds up healing. But don't apply too much; salicylic acid can temporarily dry out the skin.

Benefits of AHAs and BHA	Guidelines
Encourages skin exfoliation*	Improvement within 28 days
Increases epidermal thickness**	Best results with long-term use; can use an AHA peel product once weekly for maintenance
Improves elastic fibers (longer, thicker, less fragmented)**	Suitable for most skin types (dry to oily skin)
Increases cell proliferation***	Use with caution because peeling and redness can occur
Increases collagen production***	Don't apply to eczema or very sensitive skin
Promotes a softer and smoother skin texture	Don't use BHA if you are allergic to aspirin or salicylates
Reduces fine lines and wrinkles	Glycolic acid may increase wrinkles if overused (limit to once weekly); lactic acid and malic acid are gentler, with hydrating properties — ideal for dry and aging skin
Treats dry and rough skin	
Reduces blemishes and acne	
Reduces blackheads	
Reduces pigmentation and discoloration	

* Treatment with 4% glycolic acid applied twice daily for 3 weeks to healthy humans.

** Treatment with 15% glycolic acid for 6 months on the facial skin of postmenopausal women.

*** Cultured human skin fibroblasts were treated for 24 hours with glycolic acid and malic acid. The ranges of cell proliferation and collagen production were significantly higher with glycolic acid treatment than with malic acid or placebo.

AHAs may be listed as glycolic acid, lactic acid, or malic acid, and research shows that 5% to 15% concentrations offer best results. For BHA in skin care, look for the ingredient salicylic acid — 1% to 2% concentrations are effective. Products containing more than 8% AHAs or BHA are sold by dermatologists, laser clinics, beauticians, and cosmetic physicians, and they can also be given in the form of chemical peels.

AHAs and BHA can cause the skin to temporarily peel, flake, and look inflamed, which is to be expected, but this can often be avoided by using lactic acid or malic acid instead of glycolic acid and by applying the product sparingly. Most products sold in cosmetic department stores have only 4% or less AHA/BHA. Refer to online product review websites.

3. Resveratrol

Resveratrol, a unique antioxidant present in the skin of red grapes, red wine, blueberries, mulberries, and cranberries, has an impressive range of anti-aging properties. Dietary resveratrol significantly inhibits AGE formation, and research studies show it has the ability to block chemically induced skin cancers from forming.

The role of resveratrol in skin-care products has been of much interest to researchers because resveratrol-based skin-care formulations show 17 times greater antioxidant activity than ones containing idebenone — a popular ingredient that is closely related to coenzyme Q10. Because it has shown signs of blocking skin cancers from forming, the research on resveratrol has sparked the interest of skin-care manufacturers, who are now using the ingredient in moisturizers and sunscreens — in addition to standard UV blockers, such as zinc oxide.

> Dietary resveratrol significantly inhibits AGE formation, and research studies show it has the ability to block chemically induced skin cancers from forming.

Benefits of resveratrol	Guidelines
Has a potent antioxidant effect Reduces oxidative stress Inhibits AGE formation May reduce risk of skin cancers Is anti-inflammatory, antibacterial, antifungal, and antiviral Is a useful addition to sunscreen products	Best results with long-term use Suitable for all skin types (very dry to oily skin)

4. Vitamin C

A potent antioxidant in the skin, vitamin C (ascorbic acid) promotes collagen production and enhances the skin repair process. UV sunlight depletes the level of vitamin C in the skin, and topical products containing antioxidants can help to replenish the skin and boost daily protection against UV rays.

Vitamin C in skin-care products may be listed as ascorbic acid, L-ascorbate, or ascorbyl palmitate. Refer to online product review websites.

Benefits of vitamin C	Guidelines
Promotes collagen production	Use daily in the morning
Reduces wrinkle formation	Best results with long-term use
Boosts effectiveness of vitamin E	May cause irritation in sensitive skin; do not apply over rosacea, acne, eczema, or rashes
Speeds wound healing and repair	
Stimulates dermal fibroblasts for synthesis of collagen	Ascorbic acid is unstable in water-based products, so products usually have a short shelf life
Reduces UV/sun damage	
Reduces skin pigmentation over long term	Mix pure L-ascorbic acid crystals with moisturizer before application to ensure potency

5. Zinc Oxide and Other Sunscreen Filters

Ultraviolet sun damage is the biggest threat to younger skin, so it's essential to follow a skin-care regimen that offers protection from the sun's rays. One of the best sunscreen filters is zinc oxide because it guards against UVB and UVA sun damage. Topical products containing zinc oxide can also accelerate wound healing and repair skin cells, and zinc creams lock in moisture during the wound-healing process (and it's a common ingredient in calamine lotion and diaper rash creams). Zinc oxide can have a drying effect on the skin, so it is most suitable for normal to oily skin types.

Benefits of zinc oxide	Guidelines
Treats skin rashes Reflects UV rays Protects against sun damage Reduces risk of premature wrinkles Can reduce skin pigmentation with long-term use Assists wound healing	Apply sunscreen daily to face, hands, neck, and chest/décolletage Use mineral makeup or moisturizers with a sun protection factor (SPF) of 30 or higher (SPF 15 is not high enough) Look for sunscreen that is labeled "broad spectrum" Suitable for most skin types; if you have very dry skin, zinc oxide may make your skin feel drier

For those who cannot use liquid sunscreens due to breakouts, there are sunscreens in mineral powder form. Refer to online product review websites.

FAQ

Q. Is Vitamin D useful for skin care?

A. Vitamin D is manufactured in the skin after direct sunlight exposure. It is also obtained through your diet. It's a fat-soluble vitamin that directly and indirectly controls more than 200 genes, so it's important your skin makes enough of it. Sunscreens block the production of vitamin D, and although your face, hands, neck, and chest should be protected with sunscreen at all times when outdoors, give your body some early-morning sun exposure before applying sunscreen. About 10 minutes of direct sunlight in the morning or later in the afternoon, when the sun is not at its hottest and most damaging, is enough to boost vitamin D production in the skin.

Also eat vitamin D–rich foods, such as fish and other seafood. Vitamin D deficiency symptoms are listed on page 112.

Special Skin-Care Ingredients

The following is a list of ingredients that are useful in general skin-care products, such as cleansers, hand creams, body lotions, liquid hand soaps, and body washes.

Apple Cider Vinegar

Apple cider vinegar is an effective disinfectant, helps to restore the acidic pH to the skin, and treats dandruff.

Apple cider vinegar is an effective disinfectant, helps to restore the acidic pH to the skin, and treats dandruff (add a splash to your shampoo along with a dash of tea tree oil to make a dandruff remedy). Add a teaspoon (5 mL) of apple cider vinegar to a bowl of water and use as a facial wash to restore pH, or add 2 tablespoons (30 mL) to bathwater for a pH-balancing bath. Note that apple cider vinegar is acidic, so make sure you dilute it before use.

Black Currant Seed Oil

Rich in gamma-linolenic acid (GLA) and omega-3, black currant seed oil is anti-inflammatory and has moisturizing properties. It is suitable for dry, irritated, and sensitive skin conditions (but not for oily or acne-prone skin). Refer to online product review websites.

Calendula

An anti-inflammatory and calming ingredient, calendula stimulates the production of collagen.

Evening Primrose Oil

Evening primrose oil contains gamma-linolenic acid (GLA), which is anti-inflammatory. It is suitable for dry skin conditions and inflamed skin prone to eczema.

Green Tea

Green tea contains polyphenols that can suppress some forms of UV-induced skin cancers.

> Green tea contains polyphenols that can suppress some forms of UV-induced skin cancers.

Lecithin

A natural emulsifier and humectant with moisturizing properties, lecithin attracts moisture to the skin and is a natural part of skin-cell membranes. It's used in many skin-care products.

Vitamin E (D-Alpha Tocopherol)

A potent antioxidant to protect skin against free radicals, vitamin E also protects skin-care products from free radical formation. Vitamin E is in most moisturizer products. Avoid synthetic vitamin E, which is identifiable by "dl" in the name (dl-alpha tocopherol).

Caution

100% vitamin E oil can cause hyperpigmentation (unattractive browning of the skin) if you use it over scars or directly on the skin. This does not occur in skin-care products with added vitamin E — problems only occur with the pure oil. Don't use a combination of vitamin E and selenium because there is an increased risk of hyperpigmentation (also avoid oral supplements of combined selenium and vitamin E). It's interesting to note that 100% vitamin E oil nearly made the list of Top Skin-Care Ingredients to Avoid because of its potential to cause hyperpigmentation.

Q. What skin-care products do you recommend?

A. This is the question I am asked the most. Please note some skin-care products containing high levels of active ingredients need to be prescribed or purchased from a doctor, dermatologist, laser clinic, beautician, or cosmetic physician, but there are some over-the-counter/online options, too. For those who prefer chemical-free products, look for skin-care products that are natural or mostly natural and free of parabens, sodium lauryl sulfate (SLS), and artificial fragrance. To find these products in your area, see Resources, page 234.

Because some skin-care products can be expensive, it can be helpful to read consumer product reviews online before you buy. You also can test the products in-store or request product samples from the manufacturer, if available. If you are fussy about chemical ingredients, check the list of ingredients of a particular product before you buy — these are usually listed online. Remember that everyone's skin is different and it's often a case of trial and error until you find the perfect match for you. But keep looking — the right skin-care products can really make a difference to your skin.

Top Skin-Care Ingredients to Avoid

There are many skin-care ingredients to avoid if you prefer natural or organic products, but this list includes the top two — chosen above all others because they can enhance the aging effect.

Sodium Lauryl Sulfate (SLS)

SLS damage can be seen under a microscope for up to 4 weeks after use, and for 9 days by the naked eye.

Sodium lauryl sulfate is the most widely researched skin-care irritant and it's often used to purposely damage the skin's protective barrier function in experiments. SLS damage can be seen under a microscope for up to 4 weeks after use, and for 9 days by the naked eye. Products containing SLS create poor skin barrier function, causing excess water loss from the skin and making it easier for other chemicals, dust mites, and bacteria to penetrate the skin. SLS can cause reactions such as rashes, dandruff, hair loss, and dry skin. It can also cause rebound oily skin and enlarged pores.

SLS is found in many foaming toiletries, such as commercial toothpastes, shampoos, cleansers, hand washes, and bubble baths — in most products that bubble and foam. Similar problematic ingredients are:

- Sodium C14-16 olefin sulfonate
- Sodium laureth sulfate — often in baby products!
- TEA-lauryl sulfate

Look for products that are sulfate-free or SLS-free — there are many at health food shops and they are becoming increasingly popular in supermarkets and other retail outlets.

> SLS can cause reactions such as rashes, dandruff, hair loss, and dry skin. It can also cause rebound oily skin and enlarged pores.

FAQ

Q. I'm on a budget and I can't afford to buy lots of skin-care products. What do you suggest?

A. If you can add only a couple of super anti-aging products to your routine, I'd suggest a daily face moisturizer with added retinol. This is a good long-term investment for your skin, with a treatment containing high-dose AHAs to encourage cell turnover and collagen production. And use any type of sunscreen that is SPF 20 or higher (sun protection is most important, so anything is better than nothing). A cheap body moisturizer, as long as it is antioxidant-rich, will help guard against oxidative damage, aging, and sun damage.

Petroleum Jelly

Petroleum jelly (petrolatum) was first discovered in the 1800s in some of America's first oil rigs; however, today's petroleum jelly is more refined and a vastly improved product. It is often recommended to combat painful, dry skin conditions and to seal in moisture for skin conditions such as eczema or psoriasis. It is fine to use sparingly on the body for these conditions.

However, this ingredient poses a number of problems for the skin on your face. Facial use of petroleum jelly can make you look older because it enlarges pores around your nose, causes rebound excessive dryness after you stop using it, and it visibly increases the growth of facial hair. Once you have increased facial hair growth, it may not be reversible — but if this occurs, speak to a beautician for advice. Waxing or laser treatment are options.

Avoid using Vaseline and papaya ointment (the petroleum varieties) as moisturizers, and avoid any skin-care products that have a jelly-like consistency (check ingredients and online reviews).

FAQ

Q. I have very dry and sensitive skin. Vitamin A and AHAs cause irritation. What should I use?

A. Products containing retinol, glycolic acid, or salicylic acid may initially cause irritation, so avoid them if you have sensitive skin. If you have a reaction, remove the product and apply a heavy-duty dry skin moisturizer over the top. Also look for skin-care products that are specially formulated for dry and sensitive skin. Read skin-care reviews online and if possible test products before purchase.

Skin-Care Regimen

Now that we've discussed the best and worst ingredients to look out for in skin-care products, let's look at your morning and evening skin-care regimens.

Morning Face Care Ritual

1. Rinse face and neck with water. Cleanse with only a gentle skin cleanser if necessary; you don't want to wash away your skin's protective oils too often.

2. Optional: if you have blemishes, sparingly apply a BHA/salicylic acid product to the affected areas; or if you have hyperpigmentation, apply a lightening product or AHA product to the affected area or areas.

3. Apply face moisturizer with added vitamin C.

4. Put on sunscreen or mineral makeup with SPF 20 or higher.

FAQ

Q. I have eczema and my skin is frequently irritated. Is this 28-day program right for me?

A. If you have eczema, multiple food sensitivities, skin rashes, or irritated skin, this program may be unsuitable for you, especially while you are experiencing flare-ups. It would be better for you to begin with the program detailed in my book *The Eczema Diet*. After your eczema has improved, you can begin the 28-day program for younger skin. See Resources, page 234, for more information.

Morning Body Care Routine

1. Apply body moisturizer (one with added antioxidants) after showering.

2. Apply sunscreen to hands, neck, and chest if not covered by clothing.

3. Other parts of the body need 10 minutes of direct sunlight exposure to produce vitamin D in the skin. Afterward, if you are spending long periods in the sun, apply sunscreen to the rest of your body.

Evening Face Care Ritual

1. Cleanse skin and remove makeup (a good cleanser should not make the skin feel tight or dry — if it does, the product is too harsh).

2. Apply moisturizer with added retinol (begin with low-dose retinol with added antioxidants, or use every second night if you have sensitive skin).

Additional Face Care

- Once weekly, use an AHA product to exfoliate the skin. Refer to the AHA section on page 118.

Evening Body Care Routine

1. Shower if desired.

2. If you have aged hands, neck, or chest, apply a serum, moisturizer, or treatment containing retinol, vitamin C, or AHAs. Alternatively, apply a general body moisturizer that contains antioxidants.

Additional Body Care

- Once weekly, do a foot soak and scrub or exfoliate the feet with a pumice stone in the shower.
- Once weekly, exfoliate your body using an exfoliating mitt and a gentle body wash.

Did You Know?

Exfoliation Guidelines

It is not absolutely essential to exfoliate, but if you have dry skin, flaky skin, blackheads, wrinkles, or premature aging, or if you need to remove the last remnants of a fake tan, then a granulated cream or a quick scrub will leave your body or face looking and feeling softer and visibly smoother. However, you must take care not to use harsh exfoliators that can scratch the delicate skin on your face.

Exfoliating removes dead skin cells that tend to look flaky and dry, leaving your skin looking more smooth and hydrated.

Exfoliating Your Skin

There are several types of exfoliators for the skin: AHA products, exfoliation mitts, dry-skin brushes (a long-handled brush that enables you to reach your back), and exfoliating scrubs — creams or gels that contain granules or beads. These microscopic beads "polish" the skin as you rub them in a circular motion and are most commonly used in face-exfoliating products.

Exfoliating removes dead skin cells that tend to look flaky and dry, leaving your skin looking more smooth and hydrated. Your skin may be a little red afterward, especially if you have sensitive skin — so be gentle. The best time to exfoliate is at night, before bed; any skin redness will subside during sleep.

Alpha-hydroxy acid (AHA) products not only exfoliate the skin, with long-term use, they also trigger collagen renewal and can reduce enlarged pores and blackheads. AHA products may not be suitable if you have sensitive skin. Always remember to use sunscreen products during the day if AHAs are a part of your skin-care routine.

If you have sensitive skin and would like to use a facial exfoliator, choose one with spherical beads; they are gentler than ones made from apricot kernels. For the body, you can use mitts, natural body scrubs, or dry-skin brushes. Don't forget to exfoliate your knees, knuckles, elbows, and feet.

However, don't exfoliate your skin if you have acne; doing so may spread pimples. And avoid exfoliating broken skin, such as wounds, bites, or rashes (for example, eczema).

> Avoid exfoliating broken skin, such as wounds, bites, or rashes (for example, eczema).

How to Use a Body Exfoliator

1. Have a quick shower.
2. Spread a generous amount of scrub onto your damp skin — or use an exfoliating mitt (which feels like Velcro) with a gentle non-SLS body wash.
3. Massage with circular motions. Start at the feet and work your way up toward the heart (this is also how you use the exfoliator mitts).
4. Exfoliate from your hands to your shoulders, to your chest, and do as much of your back as possible (a dry-skin brush is useful for exfoliating the back).
5. Rinse thoroughly with water (by showering) and then moisturize. Your body should feel deliciously soft!

Body Wash

To protect your skin's acid mantle, use gentle body washes, hand washes, and cleansers that are pH balanced or that contain acidic ingredients, such as lemon or apple cider vinegar. Product labels will outline if the product is pH balanced. Look for gentle liquid soaps that are SLS- or sulfate-free.

Health food shops usually have suitable products; ask for assistance if you need advice. Add a tiny amount of apple cider vinegar to your hand- and body-wash products at home — less than a teaspoon (less than 5 mL) will do.

Buy a pumice stone from the pharmacy and use it weekly to exfoliate your feet in the shower — it's so important to scrub your feet, and pumice stones are the best.

Foot Soak and Scrub

Feet are often neglected and they can develop all types of unattractive problems later in life, such as cracked heels and hard calluses. To remove dead skin, minimize calluses, and have younger, more beautiful feet, follow the routine outlined below at least once a week. If you don't have time, buy a pumice stone from the pharmacy and use it weekly to exfoliate your feet in the shower — it's so important to scrub your feet, and pumice stones are the best. Read the notes before you begin.

You will need:

- Warm water
- Large, wide foot bowl
- 1 to 2 tablespoons (15 to 30 mL) apple cider vinegar
- Towel
- Pumice stone (one that is new and not shared with other family members)
- Foot/hand or body moisturizer

1. Place warm water into foot bowl and add vinegar.
2. Place the bowl on a towel on the floor near a chair where you can comfortably sit and soak your feet for 5 minutes.
3. Use the pumice stone, rubbing it on the soles of your feet in a circular motion. Concentrate on the hard, callused areas, but don't overdo it the first time.
4. Wash your feet and dry them.
5. Apply moisturizer (if there is a risk of slipping, you might need to wipe off the excess before walking, or avoid moisturizing the bottoms of your feet).

Note

If you have tinea or any infection on your feet or nails, treat the condition before you use a pumice stone. Otherwise, you may contaminate the pumice stone and you will need to buy a new one if this occurs.

Makeup for Younger Skin

The use of cosmetics dates back to 1200 BC, when the ancient Egyptians (who had versions of most of today's makeup products) used it to enhance facial attractiveness. Researchers at Harvard University found that women feel more confident when wearing makeup. It can increase people's perceptions of a woman's warmth, competence, and trustworthiness, and can make a woman appear younger — provided the makeup is not overdone or poorly applied.

There are exceptions to every generalization, however, and some women look more attractive without makeup — and some don't like using cosmetics, and that is fine, too. If you like using makeup, here are some tips for a younger, more flawless finish.

Primer

Applied after moisturizer, a liquid primer fills crevices and helps concealer and foundation to glide on seamlessly for a flawless finish and a more youthful appearance.

To use, wash your hands (to remove any bacteria) and apply primer to one area of your face at a time. While it is still wet, apply concealer on your problem spots and blend it in. Avoid putting too much around your eyes because it may cause your makeup to run. Primers can cause next-day breakouts if you are prone to them, and they are often filled with artificial chemicals. An alternative is to use your regular moisturizer as a primer, just before applying your makeup. If a breakout occurs from primer use, discontinue, and avoid silicon-containing primers.

Concealer

A concealer product can be used to hide dark circles under the eyes, blemishes, and hyperpigmentation. Use concealer sparingly after primer, avoid using over wrinkles, and favor products that are lightweight. If you have red patches, use a green corrector concealer, blend, and cover with a sheer powder mineral makeup — remember, less is more.

> ### Did You Know?
> **Eye Makeup**
> Unless you are a pro at applying eye shadow, keep your eye makeup simple. You will need two basics: an eyelash curler to "open up" the eyes and a lash-extending mascara — only in black. Replace your mascara frequently — every 2 months — because bacteria can build up over time.

Did You Know?

Natural Light

Before buying a makeup product, apply some from a tester and then go outside and look at your skin in natural light to check if the product matches your skin tone and looks natural. Always do your makeup in good or natural light and recheck your makeup once you are out of the house (such as when you are in your car) to see if it has been applied correctly.

Foundation

Foundation makes you look younger if it's not too obvious. It improves facial symmetry and evens out skin texture and tone.

A foundation should be used sparingly, as a concealer, or very lightly. You do not want to look as if you are wearing a mask. Poorly applied foundation can accentuate your wrinkles, so apply less and avoid foundations that have either too much shimmer or are too matte. If applying liquid foundation, use a flat, square makeup brush that doesn't soak up (and waste) your makeup. Apply to your face and partway down your neck (if the color is perfectly matched to your skin) and blend well. Reduce the shine with blotting paper or a tissue, or sparingly use powder applied with a quality mineral makeup brush.

Bronzer

Powdered or liquid bronzers are used to darken the face and neck, and to even out skin tone. However, bronzing products can make people look older (much older!) and they can go on patchy if you have dry, rough, or wrinkled skin. If you are over the age of 30, it is often best to avoid bronzers or, if necessary, apply them sparingly — to give your skin a hint of "natural" color (rather than an artificial tanned look).

Quality bronzing powder is best used to even out the skin tone: for example, use it on your neck if it needs darkening to match the tone of your face, or if you have patchy skin that needs evening out. Remember, less is best. Also avoid using fake tan on your face; it can dry out the skin and accentuate wrinkles. If you are fair-skinned, your face should be slightly lighter than your body to give the appearance of younger skin.

Lipstick

French researchers found that wearing lipstick can make women appear healthier. However, avoid brown or dull-colored lipsticks, avoid shimmer tones and high gloss (unless you are under 25), and enlist the advice of an expert about color choice for your skin type. How you apply the lipstick is very important; a bumpy lip line can make you look a little disheveled.

Lipstick often goes on smoother if you first apply a small amount of liquid foundation to your lips, blend it out toward the skin around your mouth until it is almost invisible, and then blot with a tissue. This will reduce the risk of the lipstick bleeding into any nearby wrinkles, and it gives you a blank canvas to work with. Ensure the lip line is perfect by using a lipstick brush to apply the lipstick (this is the best choice) or alternatively use a matching pencil to outline. If your lipstick starts caking later in the day, wipe it off, repeat the foundation step (which will help lipstick more effectively "stick" to your lips), and reapply.

Face Steaming to Relax the Face

The face holds tension, and muscle contractions can, over time, contribute to wrinkles. It can help to consciously relax your face daily, and steaming your face before bed can also be beneficial (it can help promote a more restful night's sleep, too).

You will need:

- Large bowl (or use the basin, provided it is clean)
- Very warm water
- Small splash of apple cider vinegar (optional)
- Large, clean cotton cloth or facecloth

1. After cleaning your face and rinsing off the cleanser, fill a bowl with very warm water.
2. Add a small amount of apple cider vinegar. The vinegar is an optional step that is designed to help restore the acid mantle of the skin.
3. Wet your cloth and quickly wring out the excess water.
4. Hold the cloth against your face and gently press, imagining your facial muscles relaxing each time you breathe out.
5. Hold the cloth over your face for 5 to 10 seconds and repeat the process three times.

Part 2

The 28-Day Program

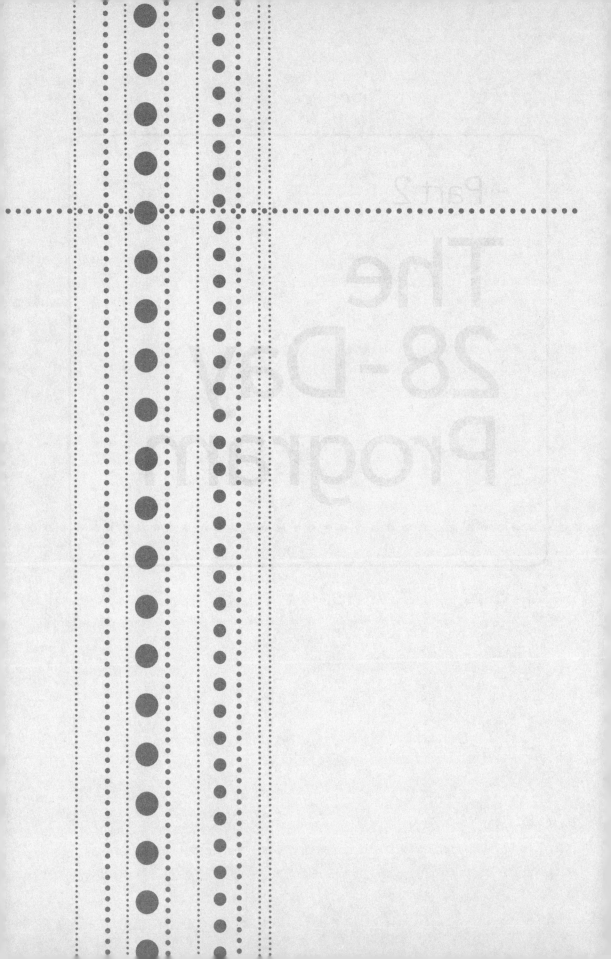

Part 2

The
28-Day
Program

Chapter 8

How This Program Works

· ·

L et's review what we have learned about skin health and skin care to create a program for achieving younger skin. This works by incorporating each of the following five factors into your daily routine. Each one helps the other to work more effectively.

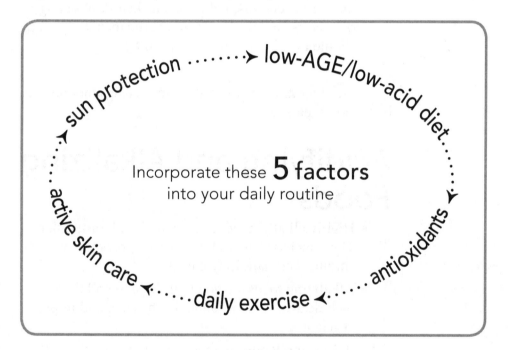

Incorporate these **5 factors** into your daily routine

sun protection ⟶ low-AGE/low-acid diet

active skin care

daily exercise

antioxidants

1. Low-AGE/ Low-Acid Diet

When combined, a low-AGE diet and a low-acid (or increased-alkaline) diet offer you the best chance at creating younger skin. The average Western diet is rich in acid-promoting foods and AGEs, and both cause premature aging of the skin.

AGEs in Your Diet

- Examples of foods that are **very low** in AGEs are whole grains, rice, tea and herbal teas, raw vegetables, and most fruits.

- Examples of **low to medium** dietary AGEs are grilled vegetables, coconut milk, raw fish (sushi), veggie burgers, and chicken or fish that has been marinated, poached, or steamed with a little lemon.

- **High** dietary AGEs are found in skinless chicken and most cooked fish — the recipes in this book will show you how to reduce the AGE content of these foods.

- **Very high** dietary AGEs are found in butter, margarine, cheeses, red meat, chicken skin, sausages, deli meats, and bacon. These are the main foods you should avoid during the 28-day program.

A list of foods containing AGEs in varying amounts can be found on page 32.

Acidifying and Alkalizing Foods

- **Highly alkalizing** foods are wonderful for the skin. These include lemon, lime, beets, apple cider vinegar, sprouts, and dark leafy greens.

- **Alkalizing** foods are good for the skin and these include avocado, raw almonds, banana, and most vegetables.

- **Acidifying foods** are fine to eat in moderation. Examples include whole grains, most fruits, most seafood, tofu, chicken, legumes, and cooked tomato.

- **Highly acidifying** foods — such as beef, pork, processed junk food, sugar, white bread, deli meats, margarine, soft drink/sodas, and alcohol — should be avoided during the 28-day program.

A list of alkalizing and acidifying foods can be found on pages 76–79.

The menus and recipes in this book show you how to shop for and prepare foods that are lower in AGEs and are acid–alkaline balanced. The recipes also show how you can lower AGEs by marinating meats and by cooking with liquids and lower temperatures.

The diet works together with the next four factors to create younger skin.

FAQ

Q. What are the main foods to avoid during the 28-day program?

A. The main foods and beverages to avoid during the 28-day program — and for younger skin — include: dairy products, wheat, refined sugar, alcohol, and red meat. If you have been diagnosed with an iron deficiency, you can add lean lamb to your diet as prescribed by your doctor (lamb is lower in AGEs and has a lower acid-producing effect than beef).

Other foods to avoid are artificial additives, most cooking oils, and margarine. I also recommend you avoid grapefruit and grapefruit juice; these block phase 1 liver detoxification and this causes increased chemicals, medical drugs (if taking), and hormones to stay in the blood, which can lead to skin problems (and to health complications if ingesting medications, drugs, or alcohol).

Avoid any foods and drinks that cause allergies, sensitivities, adverse reactions, or bloating. It is not a gluten-free program, but if you are allergic to gluten, there are simple adjustments you can make to the program so that it works for you. The 28-day program is designed to meet all the nutritional needs of a healthy adult. If you are allergic to a wide range of foods, if you are ill, or if you are a fussy eater, it's best to speak with a nutritionist or other health-care professional about your diet.

2. Antioxidants

Antioxidants protect against the oxidation of skin cells and they reduce AGE formation in the body. You can obtain antioxidant protection through both supplementation and foods, such as fruits, vegetables, and seeds — especially the ones that are red, purple, or black. The most important antioxidants, such as vitamin C, zinc, and anthocyanins, should ideally be obtained from your diet. Additional supplementation might be required if you have signs of deficiency — the Nutrient Deficiency Questionnaire on page 108 can help you identify possible deficiencies.

3. Exercise

Frequent exercise has a protective effect against AGE formation and it speeds up wound healing in older adults. Exercise reduces inflammation, normalizes glucose metabolism, and improves blood flow to the surface of your skin, giving your skin a natural, healthy glow. Daily exercise, enough to cause you to sweat, flushes microbes from the surface of your skin and assists with the removal of waste products from your body. It's also one of the keys to minimizing the appearance of cellulite.

> Frequent, medium-impact movement will give you glowing, healthy skin.

Exercise daily for 28 days — frequent, medium-impact movement is a vital part of this program and it will give you glowing, healthy skin.

4. Skin Care

Skin-care products that contain active ingredients do more than moisturize your skin — they also encourage cell renewal, increase GAGs (which offer support and hydration), increase the dermal matrix of skin, and minimize fine lines and wrinkles. Some active ingredients improve the skin's texture by forcing the skin to renew itself more quickly than it normally would. They work by setting

FAQ

Q. What types of exercise are best for the skin?

A. You have two aims when exercising: to sweat and to tone your muscles. Walking on a flat surface is not effective at toning and building muscle — and unless it's uphill and on a hot day, you will not sweat enough either. Unless you are injured or frail and cannot do much exercise, it is best to try some medium-impact exercise that also incorporates toning your problem areas (which are commonly the arms, stomach, thighs, and buttocks).

Best Forms of Exercise for Younger Skin:

- Soft-sand jogging/walking is ideal because the surface is unstable, which engages the stabilizing muscles. The stabilizing muscles are the smaller muscles that control balance, promote core strength, and act to keep certain parts of the body steady so that the primary working muscles can do their job properly. The result is increased toning of the skin. (The bonus is that the softer surface is kinder to your joints than jogging on hard surfaces.)
- Boxing and using weights are great for toning the arms (be careful not to jar your neck while throwing punches).
- Speak with an exercise coach or a personal trainer about your problem areas and have a program designed for you. An exercise coach can show you how to get results fast and avoid injuries along the way. Check the Internet for personal trainers, exercise classes, and fitness groups in your area. It is always best to try to find a teacher or personal trainer who has professionally accredited qualifications, so look for certification from the governing body for your chosen style of exercise.
- After having a baby, you can use a post-pregnancy workout DVD to tone problem areas, or speak with a personal trainer.

off a wound-healing response in the dermis layer of the skin, which triggers increased collagen production. Your diet works hand-in-hand to supply all the nutrients needed for this collagen-renewing process. Refer to Chapter 7 for more details.

No matter how perfect your diet or how many antioxidants you consume, it will be for naught if you don't use sun protection on the main aging zones: your face, neck, hands, and chest.

5. Sun Protection

Frequent UV exposure is the number one cause of wrinkles. Sun exposure causes the formation of AGEs in the skin, which paralyze collagen fibers and reduce skin elasticity. The sun depletes vitamin A in the skin, damages GAGs (which offer support and hydration), and triggers the appearance of MMPs, which degrade collagen and elastic fibers.

No matter how perfect your diet or how many antioxidants you consume, it will be for naught if you don't use sun protection on the main aging zones: your face, neck, hands, and chest. During the next 28 days, wear a hat and use sunscreen — they are the best anti-aging weapons. (If you don't like liquid sunscreen, there are non-liquid options, too, covered on page 121. Hat information starts on page 47.)

Did You Know?

Wear Driving Gloves

While driving, your hands are exposed to direct sunlight for long periods. Gloves serve to protect your hands from sun exposure, age spots, and wrinkled fingers. American researchers found that sunlight coming in through the driver's side of the car can contribute to skin cancer development on that side of your body. A total of 92% of skin cancers occur on the sun-exposed areas of the head, neck, arms, and hands, so protect these while driving.

Tips You Might Not Have Thought of for Younger Skin

Here are some more tips to help you look your best.

Sleep on Your Back

Researchers from Turkey studied people with oblique or horizontal wrinkles on their face and found they all had one thing in common: they slept in a prone position with their face buried in their pillow. If you find it hard to sleep on your back, hug a pillow to your chest; it promotes a secure feeling that enables your body to relax.

A study found that more than 8 hours of sleep each night can shorten your lifespan.

Don't Oversleep

For beauty sleep, enjoy 7 to 8 hours of quality sleep each night — but don't sleep for longer. Oversleeping promotes dehydrated skin. A study found that more than 8 hours of sleep each night can shorten your lifespan.

Steam Your Face Before Bed

Frown lines between the eyebrows and crow's-feet at the corners of the eyes are thought to be caused by small muscle contractions. Your face can be incredibly tense without you realizing it, and habitual facial expressions, such as squinting and frowning, eventually leave their mark. Face steaming helps to relax facial muscles and promotes better sleep, and it's described on page 133.

Dress Beautifully and Be Well Groomed

British researchers demonstrated how ill-fitting or plain clothing can age a 55-year-old woman by 7 years. In contrast, they found that a well-cut wardrobe (quality fabrics, plus stylish and well-fitting garments) sheds up to 8 years from a woman's face — that's a total of 15 years younger!

Don't Worry So Much

Stress causes the release of the stress chemical adrenaline, which inhibits proper digestion. Cortisol is also released, and it increases blood sugar levels and promotes collagen loss. The result is prematurely aged skin and frown lines between your eyebrows.

Laugh and Smile More

The faces of happy people look 3 years younger than non-smiling people, according to German researchers.

FAQ

Q. My skin has broken out. What should I do?

A. Breakouts can occur early in the program for several reasons:

1. If you are not used to eating plenty of fresh vegetables and following a cleansing diet, you may experience typical detoxification symptoms. Fatigue and breakouts can occur because your body is eliminating an increased amount of toxins. These symptoms should subside within a week. Just ensure you are drinking plenty of hydrating liquids.

2. A new moisturizer or a cleanser that is too oily or not right for your skin type can cause breakouts, and these will subside quickly with a change in products. Also avoid makeup primers and liquid sunscreens if you find they cause pimples (powdered sunscreens are an alternative, and you can use your daily moisturizer as makeup primer).

3. Active ingredients, such as AHAs and vitamin C, can cause temporary breakouts because they activate deep cleansing within the skin. Symptoms should stop within a week. However, if a product continually causes pimples, stinging, redness, or rashes, then discontinue use.

4. Stress can trigger breakouts, so seek advice on managing stress, worry, and anxiety.

5. Eating a food that is not right for your skin type can trigger breakouts in some individuals. If you are prone to acne, oily skin, or minor breakouts, reduce your intake of fats. Avoid cooking oils, rice bran oil (extra virgin olive oil may be okay in moderation), flaxseed oil, flax seeds, LSA (a mix containing ground flax seeds, sunflower seeds, and almonds), nuts (especially almonds), almond milk, and red meats (saturated fat) because they increase oil content in the skin. If breakouts occur, use skin-care products with added salicylic acid, formulated for treating pimples, and drink more water.

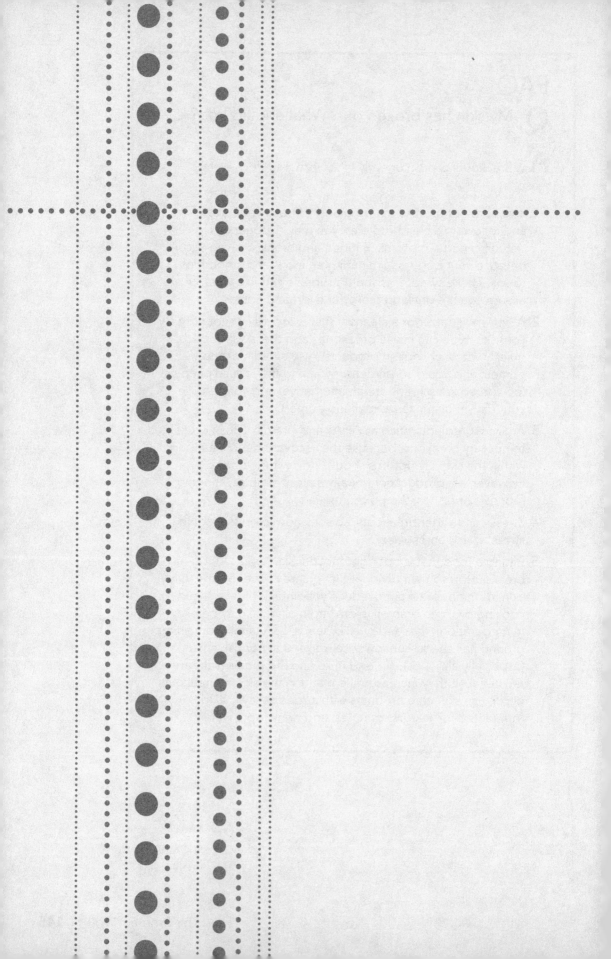

Chapter 9

The 28-Day Menu Plan

· ·

Planning meals for younger skin can be a challenge — and a delight. Here is a sample menu designed for adults with aging skin. It begins with a 3-Day Alkalizing Cleanse, where you eat foods with predominantly alkalizing ingredients to enhance liver detoxification of chemicals and to cleanse the digestive tract. It is low-AGE and really great for the skin. This food-based cleanse is a part of a 14-day meal plan that is repeated to make it a 28-day program (so you do the cleanse twice). If you are frail, unwell, pregnant, breastfeeding, or suffering from a medical condition requiring medications, you should skip the 3-Day Alkalizing Cleanse, as it is a detoxification program.

FAQ

Q. Do I need to strictly follow the 28-day menu?

A. This is a flexible program. If you have allergies or aversions, you can adapt the menus to suit your tastes and needs. You can also adjust the program to suit your skin; refer to the Quick Guide to Skin Problems and Their Treatments, which starts on page 12. If you prefer not to follow the menus, refer to the recipes in Chapter 11 and design a program to suit your tastes.

Recipes and Snacks for Your Skin Type

The following table lists the recipes included in Chapter 11, as well as some general snack options. Next to each recipe you will find a guide to which skin types the recipe is most suitable for. Note that when it says "normal to very dry skin," this means the recipe contains ingredients that boost the sebum and moisture content of the skin; it may not be suitable for people with oily or blemish-prone skin.

Recipes	Suitable for which skin types?
Breakfasts and Beverages	
Omega Muesli	All skin types
Berry Porridge	All skin types
Quinoa Porridge	Normal to very dry skin
Perfect Poached Eggs	All skin types
Boiled Eggs	All skin types
Scrambled Eggs with Watercress	All skin types
Almond Milk	Dry to very dry skin
Banana, Lemon and Coconut Smoothie	Normal to very dry skin
Moisture Boost Smoothie	Dry to very dry skin
Flaxseed Lemon Drink	Normal to very dry skin
Cucumber and Mint Juice	All skin types
Green Glow Juice	All skin types
Purple Carrot Juice	All skin types
Dandelion Tea	All skin types
Chai Tea with Clove	All skin types
Lemon and Ginger Tea	All skin types
Lemon and Mint Tea	All skin types
Green Water	All skin types
Lunch and Dinner	
Anti-Aging Broth	All skin types
Watercress Soup	All skin types
Spiced Sweet Potato Soup	All skin types
Shiitake Vegetable Soup	All skin types
Chicken and Barley Soup	All skin types
Mediterranean Seafood Soup	All skin types
Guava and Arugula Salad	All skin types
Mango and Black Sesame Salad	All skin types

Recipes	Suitable for which skin types?
Beet and Carrot Salad	All skin types
Sweet Potato Salad	All skin types
Quinoa and Pomegranate Salad	All skin types
Mixed Salad Wrap	All skin types
Shiitake Vegetable Casserole	All skin types
Eggplant and Cauliflower Curry	All skin types
Winter Spiced Dal	All skin types
Sushi Rolls with Black Sesame	All skin types
Parcel-Baked Fish	All skin types
Steamed Fish with Coconut and Lime Marinade	All skin types
Moroccan Lemon Chicken	All skin types
Oregano Chicken Skewers	Normal to very dry skin
Steamed Chicken and Mint Meatballs	All skin types
Spelt Flatbread	All skin types
Lemon Thyme Pizza	Normal to very dry skin
Marinades and Dressings	
Peach, Thyme and Chile Marinade	All skin types
Coconut and Lime Marinade	All skin types
Tamari, Lime and Ginger Marinade	All skin types
Tamari, Lycopene and Lemon Marinade	All skin types
Anchovy and Mustard Marinade	Normal to very dry skin
Ginger and Lime Dipping Sauce	All skin types
Anchovy and Mustard Dressing	All skin types
Halo Dressing	Normal to very dry skin
Snacks, Dips and Spreads	
Papaya Cups with Lime and Guava	All skin types
Lime and Berry Ice Pops	All skin types
Vegetable Platter	Best snack for all skin types
Avocado and Thyme Dip	All skin types
Beet and Almond Dip	Normal to very dry skin
Hummus Dip	All skin types
Almond Pesto	Dry to very dry skin
Banana Carob Spread	All skin types

continued...

Recipes	Suitable for which skin types?
Other Snack Options	
Handful of raw almonds and 2 Brazil nuts (for selenium)	Normal to very dry skin
6 oysters, once a week (for zinc, copper)	All skin types
2 to 3 pieces of fruit daily. Choose from: guavas; Kumatoes; $\frac{1}{4}$ cup (60 mL) blueberries or raspberries; 1 cup (250 mL) cherries or red seedless grapes; 1 banana, green apple, red apple (not Pink Lady), apricot, pomegranate, or peach; or $\frac{1}{2}$ mango (avoid fruits that cause bloating)	All skin types (especially acne-prone)

FAQ

Q. I'm quite thin and I don't want to lose weight; do I need to modify the program?

A. The 28-day menu can cause weight loss if you are not used to eating cleansing or healthy foods. Thin people may need to eat an extra meal each day to maintain their weight, such as Omega Muesli (page 166) for dessert. Ensure that you are consuming quality carbohydrates with each meal (rice, oats, barley, sweet potato, spelt pasta), enjoy smoothies for snacks, or add avocado to lunches.

Prepare Ahead

If you plan to eat soups or dal during the 3-day cleanse, make Anti-Aging Broth (page 184) *the day before* you start Day 1. Also presoak your quinoa the night before, to make Quinoa Porridge (page 168) on Day 1, using red quinoa instead of white. I recommend presoaking quinoa each day. If you forget, you can still make the porridge; it will just take a bit longer.

Once you move past the 3-day cleanse, you have the option of Omega Muesli (page 166) for some of your breakfasts. Whenever you plan to have oats for the next day's breakfast, soak the oats the night before.

On Days 5, 9, and 12, place two peeled bananas in the freezer so you'll have them ready for making smoothies in the upcoming days.

On Day 6, make a double batch of Lime and Berry Ice Pops (page 227) so you have them ready for the following week.

The 3-Day Alkalizing Cleanse

During the first 3 days of the 28-day program, drink plenty of filtered water and eat raw vegetables daily: carrot and celery sticks, sprouts, broccoli, mixed leaf salads. Don't go hungry — eat as much soup and as many raw veggies as you like. It is also important to rest and not go out socializing during the cleanse, as you need to avoid all other foods for 3 days, and have 7 to 8 hours of quality sleep at night.

Snacks during the cleanse include Vegetable Platter (page 228); Papaya Cups with Lime and Guava (page 226); a handful of raw almonds and 2 to 4 Brazil nuts daily.

If taking calcium and chromium supplements, have them twice a day with breakfast and lunch, or according to the manufacturer or as prescribed. If you are a woman, you need to consume about 18 mg of iron daily, so I recommend you take a natural herbal iron supplement. An iron supplement is also essential if you are vegetarian or vegan (see the food sources of iron on page 106).

FAQ

Q. During the first week, will I experience a detox effect?

A. The 3-Day Alkalizing Cleanse is designed to greatly improve the detoxification of chemicals; temporary symptoms, such as increased tiredness and changes in the skin, may occur. If you have an overgrowth of *Candida albicans*, either on the skin or in the mouth or digestive tract, you might experience irritability and tiredness, as well as increased cravings for sugar. This should pass quickly. Ensure you drink plenty of water. If you want to reduce any detox symptoms, decrease your intake of Anti-Aging Broth (page 184) and vegetable juices.

Alkalizing Drinks

For all 28 days, consume two to three alkalizing drinks daily. There are some suggestions in the menus, but after a few days you can choose your favorite drinks. Alkalizing drinks include Flaxseed Lemon Drink (page 175), Cucumber and Mint Juice (page 176), Green Glow Juice (page 177), Purple Carrot Juice (page 178), and herbal teas such as Dandelion Tea (page 179), Lemon and Ginger Tea (page 181), Lemon and Mint Tea (page 182), peppermint tea, and chamomile tea. Do not consume caffeine during the 3-day cleanse: no coffee, green tea, white tea or black tea, including chai. Refer to the recipe list on page 148 to see which drinks are most suitable for your skin type.

FAQ

Q. I am 25 years old and I already have good skin. Will I notice a difference if I follow the program?

A. If you already have young skin, you won't see dramatic results. However, the program will teach you how to care for your skin and body so that it looks its best for many years to come.

Days 1 to 3: The 3-Day Alkalizing Cleanse

Before breakfast, exercise for 30 to 60 minutes. Drink 6 cups (1.5 L) of water and two to three alkalizing drinks daily (see list, page 152).

Breakfast	Lunch	Dinner
Quinoa Porridge (page 168) Lemon and Ginger Tea* (page 181), Flaxseed Lemon Drink (page 175), Green Water* (page 182), Green Glow Juice (page 177), or Purple Carrot Juice (page 178)	*Choose from:* Sweet Potato Salad (page 195), Shiitake Vegetable Soup* (page 188), Spiced Sweet Potato Soup (page 187), or Watercress Soup (page 186)	*Choose from:* Sweet Potato Salad (page 195), Shiitake Vegetable Soup* (page 188), Spiced Sweet Potato Soup (page 187), Watercress Soup (page 186), or Winter-Spiced Dal (page 201) Papaya Cups with Lime and Guava* (page 226; 1 serving daily)

* For busy people, the fastest or easiest recipes are denoted with an asterisk.

Day 4

Before breakfast, exercise for 40 to 60 minutes. Drink 4 to 6 cups (1 to 1.5 L) of water and two to three alkalizing drinks daily (see list, page 152).

Breakfast	Lunch	Dinner
Choose from: Omega Muesli* (page 166) or Scrambled Eggs with Watercress (page 171) Tea of choice Green Water* (page 182) or Cucumber and Mint Juice (page 176)	*Choose from:* Quinoa and Pomegranate Salad (page 196) or Mixed Salad Wrap (page 198), or use up leftovers	*Choose from:* Parcel-Baked Fish (page 204) or Eggplant and Cauliflower Curry (page 200), or use up leftovers Papaya Cups with Lime and Guava* (page 226)

Day 5

Before breakfast, exercise for 40 to 60 minutes. Drink 4 to 6 cups (1 to 1.5 L) of water and two to three alkalizing drinks daily (see list, page 152).

Breakfast	Lunch	Dinner
Choose from: Berry Porridge (page 167) or Quinoa Porridge (page 168) Tea of choice Green Water* (page 182) or Green Glow Juice (page 177)	*Choose from:* Quinoa and Pomegranate Salad (page 196) or Mixed Salad Wrap (page 198), or use up leftovers **Afternoon snack:** Vegetable Platter (page 228) or fruit (berries or cherries)	*Choose from:* Moroccan Lemon Chicken (page 207) or Shiitake Vegetable Casserole* (page 199), or use up leftovers

Day 6

Before breakfast, exercise for 40 to 60 minutes. Drink 4 to 6 cups (1 to 1.5 L) of water and two to three alkalizing drinks daily (see list, page 152).

Breakfast	Lunch	Dinner
Choose from: Omega Muesli* (page 166) or Quinoa Porridge (page 168) Tea of choice Purple Carrot Juice* (page 178)	*Choose from:* Sweet Potato Salad (page 195) or Mixed Salad Wrap (page 198), or soup of choice **Afternoon snack:** Vegetable Platter (page 228) or fruit (guava, papaya, or peach)	*Choose from:* Winter Spiced Dal (page 201) or use up leftovers **Optional dessert:** Moisture Boost Smoothie (page 174) or a banana

Day 7: Treat Day

Before breakfast, exercise for 40 to 60 minutes. Drink 4 to 6 cups (1 to 1.5 L) of water and two to three alkalizing drinks daily (see list, page 152).

Breakfast	Lunch	Dinner
Choose from: Scrambled Eggs with Watercress* (page 171) or Banana, Lemon and Coconut Smoothie (page 173) Chai Tea with Clove* (page 180)	*Choose from:* Sushi Rolls with Black Sesame (page 202) or store-bought sushi, or use up leftovers **Afternoon snack:** Vegetable Platter (page 228) or fruit (berries or cherries)	*Choose from:* Mediterranean Seafood Soup (page 190) or Lemon Thyme Pizza (page 212) with a side of mixed salad leaves, or a restaurant option (see FAQ, page 84) Lime and Berry Ice Pop* (page 227) or Papaya Cups with Lime and Guava* (page 226)

Day 8

Before breakfast, exercise for 40 to 60 minutes. Drink 4 to 6 cups (1 to 1.5 L) of water and two to three alkalizing drinks daily (see list, page 152).

Breakfast	Lunch	Dinner
Choose from: Omega Muesli* (page 166) or Quinoa Porridge (page 168) Tea of choice Cucumber and Mint Juice (page 176)	*Choose from:* Quinoa and Pomegranate Salad (page 196) or Mixed Salad Wrap (page 198), or use up leftovers	*Choose from:* Steamed Chicken and Mint Meatballs (page 210) with steamed greens or a salad, or soup of choice Lime and Berry Ice Pop* (page 227) or fruit (banana or peach)

Day 9

Before breakfast, exercise for 40 to 60 minutes. Drink 4 to 6 cups (1 to 1.5 L) of water and two to three alkalizing drinks daily (see list, page 152).

Breakfast	Lunch	Dinner
Choose from: Perfect Poached Eggs (page 169) with spelt bread, Boiled Eggs (page 170), or Omega Muesli* (page 166) Tea of choice Green Water* (page 182) or Green Glow Juice (page 177)	*Choose from:* Beet and Carrot Salad (page 194) with Spelt Flatbread (page 214), Mango and Black Sesame Salad (page 193), or store-bought sushi	*Choose from:* Shiitake Vegetable Soup* (page 188) or Eggplant and Cauliflower Curry (page 200) Lime and Berry Ice Pop* (page 227)

Day 10

Before breakfast, exercise for 40 to 60 minutes. Drink 4 to 6 cups (1 to 1.5 L) of water and two to three alkalizing drinks daily (see list, page 152).

Breakfast	Lunch	Dinner
Choose from: Omega Muesli* (page 166), Quinoa Porridge (page 168), or Moisture Boost Smoothie (page 174) Tea of choice Purple Carrot Juice (page 178)	*Choose from:* Mixed Salad Wrap (page 198) or Quinoa and Pomegranate Salad (page 196)	*Choose from:* Steamed Fish with Coconut and Lime Marinade (page 206) or Spiced Sweet Potato Soup (page 187) Papaya Cups with Lime and Guava* (page 226)

Day 11

Before breakfast, exercise for 40 to 60 minutes. Drink 4 to 6 cups (1 to 1.5 L) of water and two to three alkalizing drinks daily (see list, page 152).

Breakfast	Lunch	Dinner
Choose from: Omega Muesli* (page 166) or Quinoa Porridge (page 168) Tea of choice Purple Carrot Juice (page 178)	*Choose from:* Mixed Salad Wrap (page 198) or Quinoa and Pomegranate Salad (page 196)	*Choose from:* Oregano Chicken Skewers (page 208) or Watercress Soup (page 186) Lime and Berry Ice Pop* (page 227) or Moisture Boost Smoothie (page 174)

Day 12

Before breakfast, exercise for 40 to 60 minutes. Drink 4 to 6 cups (1 to 1.5 L) of water and two to three alkalizing drinks daily (see list, page 152).

Breakfast	Lunch	Dinner
Choose from: Perfect Poached Eggs (page 169) with spelt bread, Boiled Eggs (page 170), or Omega Muesli* (page 166) Tea of choice Green Water* (page 182) or Green Glow Juice (page 177)	*Choose from:* Sweet Potato Salad (page 195) or Mixed Salad Wrap (page 198) **Afternoon snack:** Vegetable Platter (page 228)	*Choose from:* Mediterranean Seafood Soup (page 190) or use up leftovers Fruit (papaya and cherries, or sliced apple)

Day 13

Before breakfast, exercise for 40 to 60 minutes. Drink 4 to 6 cups (1 to 1.5 L) of water and two to three alkalizing drinks daily (see list, page 152).

Choose from: Omega Muesli* (page 166) or Moisture Boost Smoothie (page 174) Tea of choice Cucumber and Mint Juice (page 176)	*Choose from:* Guava and Arugula Salad (page 192), Mixed Salad Wrap (page 198), or soup of choice	*Choose from:* Chicken and Barley Soup (page 189) or use up leftovers Fruit (papaya and cherries, or sliced apple) or Moisture Boost Smoothie (page 174)

Day 14

Before breakfast, exercise for 40 to 60 minutes. Drink 4 to 6 cups (1 to 1.5 L) of water and two to three alkalizing drinks daily (see list, page 152).

Choose from: Scrambled Eggs with Watercress* (page 171) or Banana, Lemon and Coconut Smoothie (page 173) Tea of choice	*Choose from:* Sweet Potato Salad (page 195), Mixed Salad Wrap (page 198), or soup of choice **Afternoon snack:** Vegetable Platter (page 228) or fruit (berries or cherries)	*Choose from:* Shiitake Vegetable Casserole* (page 199) or Lemon Thyme Pizza (page 212) with Mango and Black Sesame Salad (page 193) Lime and Berry Ice Pop* (page 227) or Moisture Boost Smoothie (page 174)

Days 15 to 28

Repeat the 14-day menu.

FAQ

Q. What should I do after the 28-day program to keep my skin looking good?

A. To ensure that your skin stays beautiful, you can continue with several basic principles from the program. The most important ones are:

- Eat purple foods, such as blueberries and other berries, eggplant, purple carrots, and red cabbage, on most days. Or add a side of mixed purple and green salad leaves to your lunch or dinner; they are rich in chlorophyll and contribute to healthy skin. If you have a garden, plant some red lettuce, blueberries, and purple basil (whatever is most suitable for your climate or area) so you have a supply of anthocyanin-rich foods on hand.
- Eat vitamin C–rich red and orange foods, such as guavas, sweet potatoes, papayas, peaches, red and orange bell peppers, and carrots, daily.
- Use low-AGE cooking methods, such as steaming or poaching, with added lemon. Cook meats in marinades, and simmer soups and stews at reduced temperatures. Add alkalizing lemon and lime to your drinks and meals. Drink herbal teas, water, and fresh vegetable juices often.
- Exercise three to six times a week to tone the skin.
- Continue using active skin-care products and gradually increase the strength of your retinol-containing products. It may take up to a year for your skin to tolerate high-strength retinol. Wear sunscreen and a hat to protect your face, neck, chest, and hands from future sun damage. Sun care is essential for beautiful skin beyond age 40.
- For firmer, younger skin, continue to take a calcium supplement with magnesium, vitamin D, zinc, and manganese (and copper, if necessary). For blood sugar balance, take a chromium supplement or simply add a sprinkle of cinnamon when eating grains and other carbohydrates.

Because the 28-day program is balanced and healthy, it can also be followed in the long term, if desired. If you want to incorporate some new meals into your routine, a list of health food books containing suitable recipes can be found in the Resources (page 234).

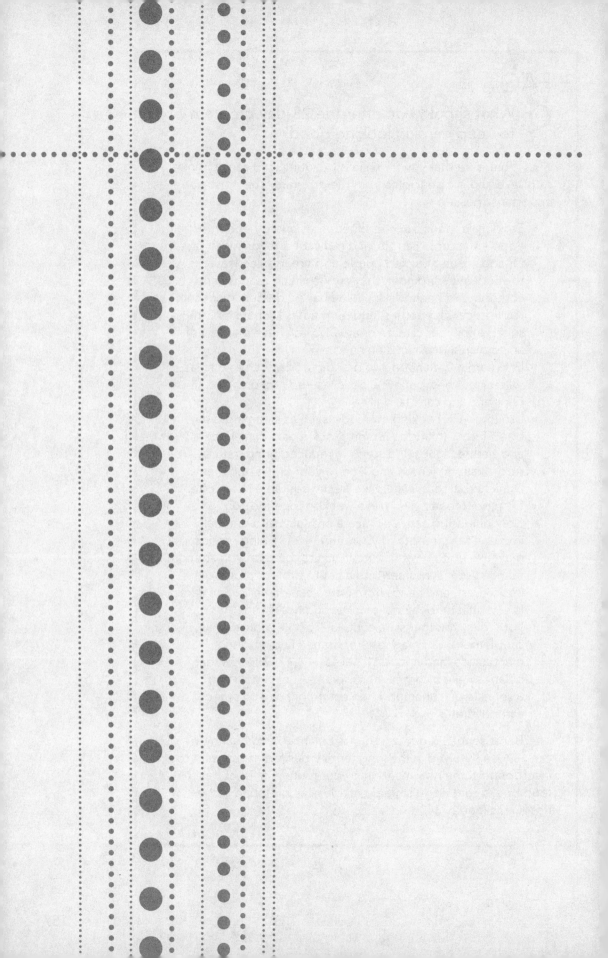

Chapter 10

Shopping List

● ●

The following shopping list covers all the ingredients you'll need to follow the 28-day menu. The amounts may vary, however, because some fresh and perishable items will need to be bought as needed and when in season (or choose seasonal alternatives). When shopping, choose products that are free of artificial additives (preservatives, colors, flavor enhancers). Remember, too, that fresh is best, and if possible choose free-range and organic products.

Guide to Symbols

* A high-use ingredient if you're following the 14-day menu
† Available in the health food section of large supermarkets and at health food shops
‡ Choose free-range or organic where possible

Fresh Produce

Perishable items, buy these weekly or as needed.

[ ] Apples, green
[ ] Asparagus
[ ] Avocados*
[ ] Bananas
[ ] Beets
[ ] Blueberries*
[ ] Broccoli or broccolini
[ ] Cabbage, red
[ ] Carrots (orange or purple)*
[ ] Cauliflower
[ ] Celery
[ ] Cherries
[ ] Cilantro, fresh*
[ ] Cucumber
[ ] Garlic
[ ] Gingerroot*
[ ] Green onions
[ ] Guava (preferably red)

[ ] Kale
[ ] Kumatoes (or plum/Roma or grape tomatoes)
[ ] Lemon thyme, fresh*
[ ] Lemons*
[ ] Limes*
[ ] Mint, fresh
[ ] Mushrooms, shiitake (or dried)
[ ] Oregano, fresh
[ ] Papaya
[ ] Parsley, fresh
[ ] Peaches
[ ] Pomegranate
[ ] Potatoes
[ ] Raspberries
[ ] Red bell peppers
[ ] Red onions*
[ ] Salad leaves, mixed (with purple leaves)*
[ ] Sprouts, mixed
[ ] Sweet potatoes*
[ ] Watercress
[ ] Zucchini

Pantry Items

[ ] Almonds, raw (not salted or roasted)
[ ] Anchovy fillets, canned
[ ] Baking soda
[ ] Bamboo skewers
[ ] Black pepper
[ ] Bouillon powder, vegetable*†
[ ] Brown rice
[ ] Brown rice flour
[ ] Carob powder
[ ] Chickpeas, dried or canned
[ ] Extra virgin olive oil (first cold pressing)*
[ ] Honey, liquid
[ ] Kombu
[ ] Lentils, dried red
[ ] Oats, rolled (not instant)*
[ ] Quinoa, red (if unavailable, buy white)†
[ ] Rice bran oil*
[ ] Rice malt syrup†

[ ] Sea salt (preferably Celtic or another quality choice)*†
[ ] Sesame seeds, black†
[ ] Spelt flour (preferably whole-grain)*
[ ] Sushi supplies (if making sushi): bamboo mat,
      sushi rice, wasabi, pickled ginger, nori sheets
[ ] Tea, chai (optional)
[ ] Tea, dandelion root (optional)
[ ] Tea, ginger (optional)
[ ] Tomato paste (preservative-free)
[ ] Vinegar, apple cider*†

Spices

[ ] Cloves, whole
[ ] Curry powder, yellow*
[ ] Garam masala*
[ ] Ground cinnamon*
[ ] Ground cumin
[ ] Hot pepper flakes (optional)
[ ] Paprika, smoked
[ ] Paprika, sweet

Fridge/Freezer

[ ] Bones for broth (2 beef, 1 to 2 chicken carcasses)‡
[ ] Calamari rings/tubes
[ ] Chicken thighs, boneless skinless*‡
[ ] Chlorophyll, liquid (optional)†
[ ] Coconut milk, light
[ ] Coconut water
[ ] Eggs (omega-3-enriched)‡
[ ] Fish (salmon, trout)*
[ ] Flaxseed oil (optional)†
[ ] Flax seeds†
[ ] Ketchup
[ ] Mustard, whole-grain
[ ] Peas, frozen
[ ] Shrimp
[ ] Soy lecithin granules (optional)†
[ ] Soy milk
[ ] Tahini (hulled tastes better)†
[ ] Tamari, reduced sodium*†

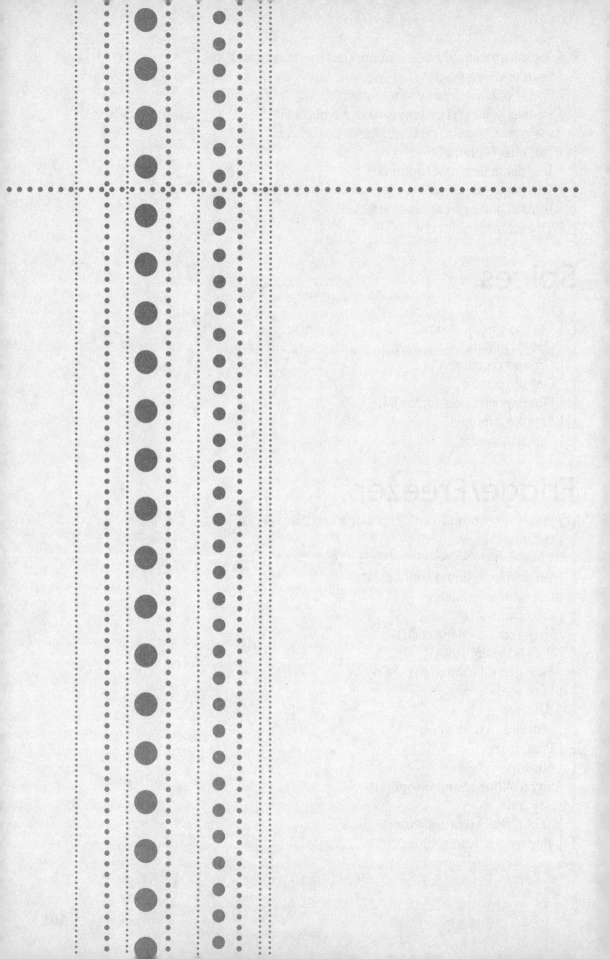

Chapter 11
Recipes

Unusual Ingredients and Substitutions

Ingredient	What is it and where do I buy it?	Substitution
Black sesame seeds	Anthocyanin-rich sesame seeds; they're not toasted but taste like it	White sesame seeds, but they don't offer the same benefit
Rice malt syrup	Natural sweetener (the only one that is alkalizing)	Agave nectar
Tahini	Paste made with sesame seeds; hulled varieties taste best	If making hummus, you can make it tahini-free by using more water, lemon juice and oil; if spreading onto bread, substitute mashed avocado
Tamari	Wheat-free and gluten-free soy sauce; choose reduced-sodium varieties with no flavor enhancers	Soy sauce (contains wheat); choose reduced-sodium varieties with no flavor enhancers

About the Nutrient Analyses

The nutrient analysis done on the recipes in this book was derived from the Food Processor SQL Nutrition Analysis Software, version 10.9, ESHA Research (2011). Where necessary, data were supplemented using the following references:

1. USDA National Nutrient Database for Standard Reference, Release #26 (2014). Retrieved February 2014, from the USDA Agricultural Research Service website: www.nal.usda.gov/fnic/foodcomp/search/.

2. Food and Drug Administration (2013). Guidance for Industry: A Food Labeling Guide (14. Appendix F: Calculate the Percent Daily Value for the Appropriate Nutrients). Retrieved February 2014, from the U.S. Food and Drug Administration website: http://www.fda.gov/food/guidanceregulation/ guidancedocumentsregulatoryinformation/ labelingnutrition/ucm2006828.htm.

Recipes were evaluated as follows:

- The larger number of servings was used where there is a range.
- Where alternatives are given, the first ingredient and amount listed were used, except for Kumatoes, where plum (Roma) tomatoes were used as a substitute.
- Optional ingredients and ingredients that are not quantified were not included.
- Calculations were based on imperial measures and weights.
- The smaller quantity of an ingredient was used where a range is provided.
- Calculations involving meat and poultry used lean portions.
- Recipes were analyzed prior to cooking.
- Nutrient values were rounded to the nearest whole number for calories, carbohydrate, protein, vitamin C, biotin and magnesium.
- Nutrient values were rounded to one decimal point for total fat, saturated fat, omega-3 fat, fiber, iron and zinc.
- Calculations for percent daily values are based on the food labeling standards set by the U.S Food and Drug Administration, which are established according to the Daily Reference Values (DRVs) and Reference Daily Intakes (RDIs) for a caloric intake of 2,000 calories for adults and children four or more years of age.

It is important to note that:

1. The cooking method used to prepare the recipe may alter the nutrient content per serving, as may ingredient substitutions and differences among brand-name products.
2. Percent daily values are based on a 2,000-calorie diet. Your daily nutrient values may be higher or lower depending on your calorie needs.

Breakfasts and Beverages

Omega Muesli

Makes 1 serving

This soaked muesli dish is rich in omega-3 and fiber. Soaking the oats and flax seeds overnight with apple cider vinegar (ACV) increases mineral availability and goodness, and it softens the oats so they can be eaten raw. Using ACV is optional, and if you forget to soak the oats overnight, just soak them for 20 minutes covered with warm water (half cool water, half boiled water from the kettle).

Tip

If you have gluten intolerance, be sure to purchase certified gluten-free oats.

¾ cup	large-flake (old-fashioned) rolled oats	175 mL
1 tsp	whole flax seeds	5 mL
	Water	
½ tsp	apple cider vinegar (optional)	2 mL
	Chilled Almond Milk (page 172), organic soy milk or water	
¼ cup	blueberries or berries of choice	60 mL
Pinch	ground cinnamon	Pinch

1. Place oats and flax seeds in a bowl with enough water to cover. Add vinegar (if using). Cover tightly with plastic wrap and leave on the counter overnight (do not refrigerate).

2. The next morning, use a strainer to drain off the water. Rinse the oats and flax seeds with water and place in a bowl. Add almond milk and top with berries and cinnamon.

Nutrients per serving	
Calories	495
Total Fat	9.7 g
Saturated Fat	1.6 g
Omega-3	1.0 g
Carbohydrate	84 g
Fiber	14.3 g (56% DV)
Protein	21 g
Biotin	23 mcg (77% DV)
Vitamin C	4 mg (7% DV)
Iron	5.8 mg (32% DV)
Magnesium	223 mg (56% DV)
Zinc	4.9 mg (33% DV)

Berry Porridge

½ cup	large-flake (old-fashioned) rolled oats	125 mL
	Water	
	Sprinkle of apple cider vinegar (optional)	
	Chilled Almond Milk (page 172), organic soy milk or water	
¼ cup	blueberries or raspberries (thawed if frozen)	60 mL
½ to 1 tsp	whole flax seeds (optional)	2 to 5 mL
Pinch	ground cinnamon	Pinch

Makes 1 serving

This hearty, warm breakfast is rich in fiber and omega-3, and has a low GI. The overnight soak is optional, but it increases mineral availability and goodness.

Tip

If you have gluten intolerance, be sure to purchase certified gluten-free oats.

1. If soaking overnight, place oats in a bowl with enough water to cover. Add vinegar (if using). Cover tightly with plastic wrap and leave on the counter overnight (do not refrigerate).

2. The next morning, use a strainer to drain off the water. Rinse the oats with water and place in a small saucepan. Add 1½ cups (375 mL) water and bring to a boil. Reduce heat to low and simmer, stirring occasionally, for 10 to 15 minutes, adding more water if necessary, until porridge is thick and oats are tender.

3. Pour the cooked oats into a bowl and top with almond milk, berries, flax seeds (if using) and cinnamon.

Nutrients per serving	
Calories	334

Total Fat
  Saturated Fat
  Omega-3
	6.2 g
	1.0 g
	0.5 g

Carbohydrate	58 g
Fiber	9.6 g (40% DV)
Protein	14 g
Biotin	16 mcg (53% DV)
Vitamin C	4 mg (7% DV)
Iron	3.9 mg (22% DV)
Magnesium	147 mg (37% DV)
Zinc	3.2 mg (21% DV)

Quinoa Porridge

Makes 1 serving

Quinoa is a nutritious gluten-free seed that cooks like a grain. Soaking the quinoa overnight is recommended to make the minerals more available, but soaking is not essential. Red quinoa contains beneficial anthocyanins and has a lower GI than white quinoa.

Tip

In place of the vanilla extract, you can use $1/2$ vanilla bean, if desired. Discard it before serving.

$1/2$ cup	red or white quinoa, rinsed (do not use puffed quinoa)	125 mL
	Water	
$1/2$ tsp	vanilla extract (optional)	2 mL
$1/2$ cup	chilled Almond Milk (page 172) or organic soy milk	125 mL
	Blueberries, papaya, banana, cherries or raspberries	
1 tsp	whole flax seeds (optional)	5 mL
Pinch	ground cinnamon	Pinch

1. If soaking overnight, place quinoa in a bowl with enough water to cover it. Cover tightly with plastic wrap and leave on the counter overnight (do not refrigerate).

2. The next morning, use a strainer to drain off the water, rinse the quinoa with water and place it in a saucepan. Add $1^1/_2$ cups (375 mL) water and bring to a boil. Reduce heat to low and simmer, stirring often, for about 15 minutes for white quinoa or 20 minutes for red quinoa, or until porridge is thick and quinoa is tender.

3. Add vanilla (if using) and milk, return to a simmer and simmer for 5 minutes, stirring occasionally to prevent burning and adding a touch more milk if necessary (you want the liquid to puff up the quinoa so it's very soft).

4. Pour the cooked quinoa into a bowl and top with fruit, flax seeds (if using) and cinnamon.

Nutrients per serving	
Calories	386

Total Fat
  Saturated Fat
  Omega-3
	11.4 g
	1.1 g
	0.5 g

Carbohydrate	57 g
Fiber	7.6 g (32% DV)
Protein	15 g
Biotin	8 mcg (27% DV)
Vitamin C	0 mg (0% DV)
Iron	4.4 mg (24% DV)
Magnesium	204 mg (51% DV)
Zinc	3.1 mg (21% DV)

Perfect Poached Eggs

<table>
<tr><td>Makes 1 to
2 servings</td></tr>
</table>

This recipe is a healthy way to cook eggs, as there is no frying involved. Eggs are a rich source of B vitamins and protein. There is an art to cooking perfect poached eggs, and these tips will turn you into a pro in no time. Serve with spelt sourdough toast and avocado, if desired.

Tip

The cooking time in step 2 may vary according to the size of the eggs and your stove's burner temperature, but after making poached eggs a couple of times, you will know what cooking time works for you.

Nutrients per 1 of 2 servings	
Calories	143

Total Fat
  Saturated Fat
  Omega-3
	9.5 g
	3.1 g
	0.1 g

Carbohydrate	1 g
Fiber	0 g (0% DV)
Protein	13 g
Biotin	20 mcg (67% DV)
Vitamin C	0 mg (0% DV)
Iron	1.8 mg (10% DV)
Magnesium	12 mg (3% DV)
Zinc	1.3 mg (9% DV)

	Water	
4 tsp	apple cider vinegar	20 mL
2	free-range large eggs	2

1. Fill a small saucepan with enough water to cover the eggs. Bring to a boil, then add vinegar (the vinegar keeps the egg whites together while cooking).

2. Remove boiling water from heat so the bubbling stops, then carefully crack the eggs into the water. Return saucepan to low heat and simmer for about $5\frac{1}{2}$ minutes for runny yolks or 7 minutes for firm yolks.

3. Carefully and swiftly remove the eggs with a slotted spoon or spatula. If desired, rinse off vinegar using slow-running hot water. Drain water off eggs and serve immediately.

Boiled Eggs

Makes 1 to 2 servings

How do you know if an egg is cooked the way you like it? Lift it out of the water with a spoon — if the shell dries immediately, the egg is hard-cooked; if it dries slowly, the yolk should be runny.

Tip
The cooking time in step 2 may vary according to the size of the eggs and your stove's burner temperature, but after making boiled eggs a couple of times, you will know what cooking time works for you.

4 tsp	white vinegar	20 mL
Pinch	salt	Pinch
2	free-range large eggs	2

1. Fill a small saucepan with enough water to cover the eggs. Bring to a boil, then add vinegar and salt (vinegar and salt help prevent the shells from cracking).

2. Gently spoon the eggs (in the shell) into the water and reduce heat to low. For runny yolks, simmer for about 3 minutes, turning eggs occasionally to promote even cooking. For firm yolks, simmer for 8 minutes.

3. Using a dessert spoon, carefully remove the eggs from the water. Place eggs briefly into cold water to halt the cooking, then peel shells, if desired. If serving soft-boiled eggs, you can place them into egg cups and cut off the top third using a knife.

Serving Suggestion
For soft-cooked eggs, sprinkle with chopped fresh parsley and serve with toast "dipping sticks" made with spelt bread. Add Kumatoes (see page 74) on the side.

Nutrients per 1 of 2 servings	
Calories	72

Total Fat
  Saturated Fat
  Omega-3
	4.8 g
	1.6 g
	0.1 g

Carbohydrate	0 g
Fiber	0 g (0% DV)
Protein	6 g
Biotin	10 mcg (33% DV)
Vitamin C	0 mg (0% DV)
Iron	0.9 mg (5% DV)
Magnesium	6 mg (2% DV)
Zinc	0.6 mg (4% DV)

Scrambled Eggs with Watercress

Makes 1 serving

Scrambling is a low-AGE way to serve eggs. Use quality free-range eggs and choose omega-3-rich eggs if possible. For acid–alkaline balance, serve the eggs with wilted watercress, as it is highly alkalizing and a good source of chlorophyll and calcium. Serve with Spelt Flatbread (page 214) or quality spelt sourdough bread, if desired.

2 tsp	water, divided	10 mL
1 cup	watercress, stems trimmed	250 mL
2	free-range large eggs	2
	Sea salt (optional)	

1. You can serve the watercress uncooked, if desired. If cooking the watercress, heat a nonstick skillet over medium heat. Add 1 tsp (5 mL) water and watercress, and heat briefly to wilt the watercress. Remove watercress from the pan, drain and set aside.

2. In a bowl, whisk together eggs and remaining water. Heat a nonstick skillet over medium heat, pour in egg mixture and cook, stirring almost constantly, for 1 to 2 minutes or until just set. Do not overcook — remove from heat before eggs begin to brown around the edges.

3. Place watercress on a serving plate and top with eggs. Season with salt, if desired.

Nutrients per serving	
Calories	143
Total Fat	9.5 g
Saturated Fat	3.1 g
Omega-3	0.1 g
Carbohydrate	1 g
Fiber	0 g (0% DV)
Protein	13 g
Biotin	20 mcg (67% DV)
Vitamin C	1 mg (2% DV)
Iron	1.8 mg (10% DV)
Magnesium	12 mg (3% DV)
Zinc	1.3 mg (9% DV)

Almond Milk

Makes 6 servings

Almonds are a super food for moisturizing the skin, plus they're alkalizing and a source of calcium and protein. You can use Almond Milk instead of cow's milk in smoothies, on porridge or on muesli. This recipe also has added flax seeds for omega-3 balance.

Caution

Almond milk is not suitable if you have oily skin, acne or eczema.

Tip

The leftover almond meal can be used to make Beet and Almond Dip (page 230). Or use it to make a body scrub to gently exfoliate your skin.

Nutrients per serving	
Calories	146

Total Fat
    Saturated Fat
    Omega-3
	12.5 g
	1.0 g
	0.4 g

Carbohydrate	6 g
Fiber	3.4 g (14% DV)
Protein	5 g
Biotin	15 mcg (50% DV)
Vitamin C	0 mg (0% DV)
Iron	1.0 mg (6% DV)
Magnesium	73 mg (18% DV)
Zinc	0.8 mg (5% DV)

- **Blender**

1 cup	whole raw almonds (not roasted or salted)	250 mL
5 cups	water, divided	1.25 L
1 tbsp	whole flax seeds	15 mL
Pinch	ground cinnamon	Pinch

1. Soak the almonds in 2 cups (500 mL) water overnight (highly recommended but not essential). Drain almonds and rinse.

2. In blender, combine drained almonds, remaining water, flax seeds and cinnamon. Blend on high for 30 seconds. Strain the liquid into a bowl, using a measuring cup or spatula to press the last of the liquid through the strainer. Cover and refrigerate for up to 5 days.

Banana, Lemon and Coconut Smoothie

Makes 2 servings

This thick, tropical smoothie is a delicious and refreshing drink. Bananas are a great source of fiber.

Variations

If your skin is oily, add a few mint leaves and use soy milk instead of almond milk.

If your skin is dry, add 1 tsp (5 mL) flaxseed oil or chia seeds.

- **Blender**

1	frozen banana, chopped (peel before freezing)	1
1 cup	chilled coconut water	250 mL
1 cup	chilled Almond Milk (page 172) or organic soy milk	250 mL
	Juice of ½ lemon	

1. In blender, combine banana, coconut water, almond milk and lemon juice. Blend on high until smooth.

Nutrients per serving	
Calories	149

Total Fat
  Saturated Fat
  Omega-3
	6.7 g
	0.8 g
	0.2 g

Carbohydrate	21 g
Fiber	4.6 g (20% DV)
Protein	4 g
Biotin	9 mcg (30% DV)
Vitamin C	8 mg (13% DV)
Iron	1.0 mg (6% DV)
Magnesium	82 mg (21% DV)
Zinc	0.6 mg (4% DV)

Moisture Boost Smoothie

Makes 2 servings

This alkalizing drink contains omega-3, anthocyanins and cryptoxanthin-rich papaya to reduce AGEs and hydrate dry, wrinkle-prone skin (it's not suitable if you have acne or oily skin).

Tip

Soy lecithin granules make oils easier to digest. Do not use lecithin if you are allergic to soy.

- Blender

1	frozen ripe banana, chopped (peel before freezing)	1
½ cup	frozen blueberries	125 mL
½ cup	diced papaya	125 mL
1 tbsp	fresh mint leaves	15 mL
1 tbsp	soy lecithin granules (GMO-free)	15 mL
Pinch	ground cinnamon	Pinch
1½ cups	chilled Almond Milk (page 172) or water	375 mL
2 tsp	flaxseed oil or whole flax seeds	10 mL

1. In blender, combine banana, blueberries, papaya, mint, lecithin, cinnamon, almond milk and flaxseed oil. Blend on high until smooth.

Nutrients per serving	
Calories	288

Total Fat
  Saturated Fat
  Omega-3
	21.2 g
	2.3 g
	3.1 g

Carbohydrate	27 g
Fiber	6.3 g (25% DV)
Protein	5 g
Biotin	13 mcg (43% DV)
Vitamin C	28 mg (47% DV)
Iron	1.4 mg (8% DV)
Magnesium	81 mg (20% DV)
Zinc	1.0 mg (7% DV)

Flaxseed Lemon Drink

Makes 2 to 3 servings

Over the years, I've had great feedback about this alkalizing drink, which was featured in the original *Healthy Skin Diet*. This new, simplified version is super-hydrating and helps to soften the skin. Enjoy it throughout the day or before each main meal. If you have acne or oily skin, omit the flaxseed oil.

- **Blender**

5	fresh mint leaves (optional)	5
1 tbsp	soy lecithin granules (GMO-free)	15 mL
¼ tsp	grated gingerroot	1 mL
2 cups	chilled water	500 mL
2 tsp	flaxseed oil	10 mL
	Finely grated zest and juice of ½ lemon	

1. In blender, combine mint (if using), lecithin, ginger, water, oil, lemon zest and lemon juice. Blend on high for 30 seconds or until frothy and thoroughly blended. Strain, if desired.

Nutrients per 1 of 3 servings	
Calories	61

Total Fat
  Saturated Fat
  Omega-3
	7.6 g
	1.0 g
	1.8 g

Carbohydrate	0 g
Fiber	0.0 g (0% DV)
Protein	0 g
Biotin	0 mcg (0% DV)
Vitamin C	0 mg (0% DV)
Iron	0.0 mg (0% DV)
Magnesium	0 mg (0% DV)
Zinc	0.0 mg (0% DV)

Cucumber and Mint Juice

Makes 2 servings

This alkalizing drink is designed to reduce inflammation, aid liver detoxification and promote a healthy skin glow.

- **Juicer**

4	celery stalks	4
2	medium or large cucumbers	2
1	knob gingerroot	1
$\frac{1}{2}$	bunch fresh mint	$\frac{1}{2}$
	Water	
	Apple cider vinegar	
	Juice of $\frac{1}{2}$ lemon	

1. Soak celery, cucumbers, ginger and mint in water with a splash of vinegar for 3 to 5 minutes, then drain.

2. Scrub celery and ginger, if needed. For a stronger ginger flavor, leave the skin on; for a milder taste, peel it off. Trim about $\frac{1}{2}$ inch (1 cm) off the mint stems.

3. Using the juicer, juice celery, cucumbers, ginger and mint, adding a splash of water at the end. Remove jug from juicer and stir in lemon juice.

Nutrients per serving	
Calories	38
Total Fat	0.5 g
Saturated Fat	0.1 g
Omega-3	0 g
Carbohydrate	7 g
Fiber	2.6 g (10% DV)
Protein	2 g
Biotin	0 mcg (0% DV)
Vitamin C	9 mg (15% DV)
Iron	0.7 mg (4% DV)
Magnesium	34 mg (9% DV)
Zinc	0.5 mg (3% DV)

Green Glow Juice

Makes 3 servings

Here's a highly alkalizing juice to thin the blood and give your skin a natural glow.

- **Juicer**

5	kale leaves	5
5	stalks celery	5
2	handfuls mixed sprouts	2
2	green apples	2
1/2	bunch fresh mint	1/2
	Water	
	Apple cider vinegar	

1. Soak kale, celery, sprouts, apples and mint in water with a splash of vinegar for 3 to 5 minutes, then drain.

2. Scrub celery, if needed. Trim about 1/2 inch (1 cm) off the mint stems.

3. Using the juicer, juice kale, celery, sprouts, apples and mint, adding a splash of water at the end.

Nutrients per serving	
Calories	105
Total Fat	0.8 g
Saturated Fat	0.1 g
Omega-3	0.1 g
Carbohydrate	25 g
Fiber	5.2 g (21% DV)
Protein	3 g
Biotin	2 mcg (7% DV)
Vitamin C	76 mg (127% DV)
Iron	1.4 mg (8% DV)
Magnesium	36 mg (9% DV)
Zinc	0.5 mg (3% DV)

Purple Carrot Juice

Makes 3 servings

This sweet juice is rich in AGE-reducing anthocyanins and carotenes.

Tip

If you cannot find purple carrots, use beets, red cabbage or purple kale and extra carrots. (Beets have a high GI, so add cinnamon to this drink if substituting beets. Avoid raw cabbage if you have thyroid problems.)

- **Juicer**

3	large stalks celery	3
2	purple carrots (see tip, at left)	2
2	large orange carrots	2
2	large apples (dark red, if possible)	2
½ cup	mixed sprouts	125 mL
	Water	
	Apple cider vinegar	

1. Soak celery, purple and orange carrots, apples and sprouts in water with a splash of vinegar for 3 to 5 minutes, then drain.

2. Scrub celery and carrots, if needed.

3. Using the juicer, juice celery, carrots, apples and sprouts, adding a splash of water at the end.

Nutrients per serving	
Calories	128

Total Fat
  Saturated Fat
  Omega-3
	0.6 g
	0.1 g
	0 g

Carbohydrate	32 g
Fiber	7.1 g (28% DV)
Protein	2 g
Biotin	4 mcg (13% DV)
Vitamin C	14 mg (23% DV)
Iron	0.9 mg (5% DV)
Magnesium	32 mg (8% DV)
Zinc	0.5 mg (3% DV)

Dandelion Tea

Makes 1 cup (250 mL)

Dandelion root is alkalizing, and some research indicates that it may increase phase II liver detoxification (where your liver deactivates and removes from the body chemicals, toxins, excess hormones and pesticides) by as much as 244%. Have up to 2 cups (500 mL) a day to stimulate digestion.

Tip

Make this tea weak to begin with, as it can be quite strong in flavor.

- **Enclosed tea strainer**

1 cup	boiling water	250 mL
$\frac{1}{2}$ tsp	ground dandelion root	2 mL
1 tsp	rice malt syrup or agave nectar (optional)	5 mL

1. Pour boiling water into a coffee mug. Place dandelion root in the tea strainer, dunk in the water and steep for about 5 seconds or until water is dark brown. Add rice malt syrup, if desired.

Cautions

More than 3 cups (750 mL) daily can overstimulate digestive acids.

Dandelion tea is not suitable if you suffer from stomach ulcers or heartburn.

Nutrients per 1 cup (250 mL)	
Calories	0
Total Fat	0.0 g
Saturated Fat	0.0 g
Omega-3	0.0 g
Carbohydrate	0 g
Fiber	0.0 g (0% DV)
Protein	0 g
Biotin	0 mcg (0% DV)
Vitamin C	0 mg (0% DV)
Iron	0.0 mg (0% DV)
Magnesium	3 mg (1% DV)
Zinc	0.0 mg (0% DV)

Chai Tea with Clove

Dandeli

Makes 1 to 2 servings

Chai tea is a delicious, antioxidant-rich tea that contains some caffeine thanks to the black tea. Store-bought chai tea bags usually contain black tea, cinnamon, ginger, cloves and cardamom. This brew has added ginger and cloves to boost the anti-inflammatory and anti-AGEing effect. As it contains some caffeine, do not drink it during the 3-Day Alkalizing Cleanse.

1 cup	boiling water	250 mL
1	chai teabag	1
1	slice gingerroot (or 1 ginger teabag)	1
1	whole clove	1

1. Pour boiling water into a teapot, then add the teabag, ginger and clove. Let steep for 5 minutes.
2. Strain the tea as you pour it into a teacup.

Variations

Add organic soy milk and 1 tsp (5 mL) rice malt syrup or agave nectar.

Add a squeeze of fresh lemon juice, or use a lemon and ginger teabag instead of the gingerroot.

Nutrients per 1 of 2 servings	
Calories	3

Total Fat
  Saturated Fat
  Omega-3
	0.1 g
	0.0 g
	0.0 g

Carbohydrate	1 g
Fiber	0.2 g (0% DV)
Protein	0 g
Biotin	0 mcg (0% DV)
Vitamin C	1 mg (2% DV)
Iron	0.1 mg (0% DV)
Magnesium	3 mg (1% DV)
Zinc	0.0 mg (0% DV)

Lemon and Ginger Tea

1 cup	boiling water	250 mL
1	thick wedge of lemon (scrub lemon skin before cutting)	1
1	large slice gingerroot	1
1	whole clove	1

Makes 1 serving

Tip

For sweetness, add 1 tsp (5 mL) rice malt syrup or agave nectar.

1. Pour boiling water into a coffee mug. Squeeze the lemon juice into the mug, then add the lemon wedge, ginger and clove. Let steep for 5 minutes.

2. If desired, strain before drinking.

Nutrients per serving	
Calories	12
Total Fat	0.1 g
Saturated Fat	0.0 g
Omega-3	0.0 g
Carbohydrate	3 g
Fiber	0.7 g (3% DV)
Protein	1 g
Biotin	0 mcg (0% DV)
Vitamin C	12 mg (20% DV)
Iron	0.2 mg (1% DV)
Magnesium	6 mg (2% DV)
Zinc	0.1 mg (1% DV)

Lemon and Mint Tea

1 cup	boiling water	250 mL
1	thick wedge of lemon (scrub lemon skin before cutting)	1
3	fresh mint leaves	3

1. Pour boiling water into a teapot or teacup. Squeeze the lemon juice into the pot or cup, then add the lemon wedge and mint. Let steep for 5 minutes.

2. If using a cup, remove the wedge and leaves before drinking.

Nutrients per serving			
Calories	6		
Total Fat	0.0 g	Biotin	0 mcg (0% DV)
Saturated Fat	0.0 g	Vitamin C	11 mg (18% DV)
Omega-3	0.0 g		
Carbohydrate	2 g	Iron	0.2 mg (1% DV)
Fiber	0.6 g (2% DV)	Magnesium	4 mg (1% DV)
Protein	0 g	Zinc	0 mg (0% DV)

Green Water

This dark green drink is highly alkalizing.

Tip
Avoid "double strength" or "high concentrate" liquid chlorophyll that is blackish in color, as it may stain your teeth with long-term use.

1 tsp	liquid chlorophyll	5 mL
1	glass chilled water or mineral water	1

1. Mix chlorophyll into water and drink.

Nutrients per serving			
Calories	15		
Total Fat	0.2 g	Biotin	0 mcg (0% DV)
Saturated Fat	0.0 g	Vitamin C	0 mg (0% DV)
Omega-3	0.0 g		
Carbohydrate	4 g	Iron	0.0 mg (0% DV)
Fiber	0.0 g (0% DV)	Magnesium	3 mg (1% DV)
Protein	0 g	Zinc	0.0 mg (0% DV)

Lunch and Dinner

Anti-Aging Broth

Makes about 8 cups (2 L)

The secret to a therapeutic broth is the addition of a weak acid, such as apple cider vinegar or lemon juice, to draw out the minerals from the bones during cooking. This alkaline broth boosts liver detoxification (so it can have a detox effect), and has anti-inflammatory and immunity-boosting ingredients. Use this broth during the 3-Day Alkalizing Cleanse or as a tasty stock in casseroles and soups.

2	large beef or lamb bones, with a little meat on them (including necks, joints, marrow)	2
1	large chicken carcass (or 2 small)	1
14 cups	water (at room temperature)	3.5 L
2 tsp	apple cider vinegar or lemon juice	10 mL
2	red onions	2
2	Brussels sprouts	2
2	stalks celery	2
1	carrot	1
1	potato (use skins if not going green)	1
3 to 4	cloves garlic, minced	3 to 4
1 tsp	sea salt (preferably Celtic)	5 mL

1. Place the beef bones, chicken carcass, water and vinegar in a stockpot or very large saucepan, cover and bring to a boil. Reduce heat and simmer for 2 hours.

2. Meanwhile, chop red onions, Brussels sprouts, celery, carrot and potato into small pieces.

3. Using tongs, break apart the chicken carcass to allow more of the minerals to be extracted from the bones. Add chopped vegetables, garlic and salt. Simmer for 4 hours, or until reduced by almost half.

4. Remove the larger bones with tongs (the chicken bones should crumble when squeezed, as the acid has caused the alkaline minerals to be extracted). Place a strainer over a large bowl, then pour the broth through the strainer. Use a measuring cup or spatula to press down on the cooked meat and vegetables, squeezing out the remaining liquid. Discard bones and vegetables.

5. Pour the broth into airtight containers and refrigerate overnight. The next day, carefully lift or skim off the layer of solidified fat and discard it.

Nutrients per 1 cup (250 mL)	
Calories	38

Total Fat
  Saturated Fat
  Omega-3
	0.5 g
	0.3 g
	0.0 g

Carbohydrate	9 g
Fiber	1.7 g (7% DV)
Protein	3 g
Biotin	1 mcg (3% DV)
Vitamin C	12 mg (20% DV)
Iron	0.5 mg (3% DV)
Magnesium	16 mg (4% DV)
Zinc	0.2 mg (1% DV)

Variation

Vegan Anti-Aging Broth:
Omit the bones, add extra vegetables and reduce the cooking time to 3 hours.

Tips

If your broth is thick and jelly-like, it means it's rich in collagen.

Don't add purple vegetables to the stock or you'll end up with a purple broth.

The broth can be stored in glass jars or other airtight containers in the refrigerator for up to 1 week, or in the freezer for up to 6 months. Most of the recipes in this book use 3 cups (750 mL) broth, so measure out portions of 3 cups (750 mL) each and write the volume on the container before freezing.

Watercress Soup

Watercress is highly alkalizing and a good source of calcium, and hummus dip adds protein and a creamy texture, with a hint of tang. When choosing potatoes, favor new potatoes, as they have a lower GI than other varieties.

Tips

If you prefer, you can replace 3 cups (750 mL) of the water with Anti-Aging Broth (page 184).

For added flavor, sprinkle the soup with a little sweet paprika after stirring in the hummus dip.

Nutrients per serving	
Calories	117

Total Fat
  Saturated Fat
  Omega-3
	1.8 g
	0.3 g
	0.0 g

Carbohydrate	23 g
Fiber	3.1 g (12% DV)
Protein	4 g
Biotin	1 mcg (3% DV)
Vitamin C	25 mg (42% DV)
Iron	0.8 mg (4% DV)
Magnesium	43 mg (11% DV)
Zinc	0.6 mg (4% DV)

- **Blender or food processor**

1 tsp	garam masala	5 mL
1 tsp	grated gingerroot	5 mL
6 cups	water	1.5 L
2 tsp	vegetable bouillon powder	10 mL
2	new potatoes, peeled and diced	2
1	red onion, finely chopped	1
1	bunch (5 oz/150 g) watercress, stalks trimmed 2 inches (5 cm), 4 sprigs reserved for garnish	1
1 tbsp	freshly squeezed lemon juice	15 mL
4 tbsp	Hummus Dip (page 231) or store-bought hummus, divided	60 mL

1. In a large saucepan, over medium heat, sauté garam masala and ginger for about 1 minute or until fragrant (be careful not to burn the spices). Add water and bouillon; increase heat and bring to a boil. Add potatoes and red onion; reduce heat to low, cover and simmer for 10 minutes. Add watercress and simmer for 3 minutes. Remove from heat and let cool for 5 minutes.

2. Stir in lemon juice, then transfer to blender and purée until smooth.

3. When serving, add a dollop of hummus dip (about $1\frac{1}{2}$ tsp/7 mL) to each bowl and stir slightly to give a creamy, streaked texture. Add another dollop of hummus to the center of the soup and top with a sprig of watercress.

Spiced Sweet Potato Soup

This easy-to-prepare soup is rich in skin-loving minerals and tastes absolutely lovely. The secret ingredient is Thai red curry paste.

Tips

Thai red curry paste may contain shrimp paste, so if you're vegetarian or vegan, use 1 tsp (5 mL) yellow curry powder in its place. Be careful not to let it burn when sautéing; add a splash of water if necessary,

Store leftover red curry paste in the freezer.

If desired, top with chopped fresh herbs, such as cilantro or parsley, and serve with spelt sourdough bread.

Nutrients per serving

Calories	213

Total Fat
  Saturated Fat
  Omega-3
	1.0 g
	0.3 g
	0.1 g

Carbohydrate	46 g
Fiber	7.9 g (32% DV)
Protein	7 g
Biotin	2 mcg (7% DV)
Vitamin C	16 mg (27% DV)
Iron	2.7 mg (15% DV)
Magnesium	66 mg (17% DV)
Zinc	1.2 mg (8% DV)

- **Blender or food processor**

1½ tbsp	Thai red curry paste	22 mL
2	cloves garlic, minced	2
1	large red onion, finely chopped	1
1 tbsp	vegetable bouillon powder	15 mL
3 cups	Anti-Aging Broth (page 184) or water	750 mL
3 cups	water	750 mL
¼ cup	dried red lentils	60 mL
4	medium-large sweet potatoes, peeled and diced	4

1. In a large saucepan, over medium heat, sauté curry paste for about 1 minute or until fragrant. Add garlic, red onion, bouillon, broth and water; increase heat and bring to a boil.

2. Meanwhile, rinse lentils thoroughly in a large bowl of water, drain and remove any discolored lentils. Stir into the saucepan, along with sweet potatoes; return to a boil. Reduce heat to low and simmer for 30 minutes. Remove from heat and let cool for 5 minutes.

3. Using a blender or food processor, blend the soup in batches to make a smooth soup. If the soup is too thick, add ½ cup (125 mL) water.

Shiitake Vegetable Soup

Makes 4 servings

Shiitake mushrooms are rich in antioxidants, including selenium and vitamins A, E, C and D. They have been used as a medicinal food for centuries and are well known for their anti-tumor properties and for lowering blood pressure, strengthening the immune system against viruses and improving liver function (which is important for healthy skin). But if you don't like shiitake mushrooms, swap them for ½ cup (125 mL) finely diced eggplant — another vegetable packed with antioxidants (in its skin).

2	stalks celery, finely chopped	2
1	red onion, finely chopped	1
1	carrot, diced	1
1 tsp	grated gingerroot	5 mL
1 tbsp	vegetable bouillon powder	15 mL
5 cups	water	1.25 L
3 cups	Anti-Aging Broth (page 184) or water	750 mL
¼ cup	sliced shiitake mushroom caps	60 mL
1 tbsp	finely chopped fresh parsley	15 mL
1 tbsp	freshly squeezed lemon juice	15 mL

1. Place celery, red onion, carrot, ginger, bouillon, water and broth in a stockpot or large saucepan, cover and bring to a boil. Reduce heat to low and simmer for 10 minutes.

2. Add mushrooms and simmer for 5 minutes or until vegetables are softened. Remove from heat and stir in parsley and lemon juice.

Tip

You can use dried shiitake mushrooms in place of fresh. Soak ¼ cup (60 mL) in a bowl of warm water for about 5 minutes, then drain before adding to the soup in step 2. Chop drained soaked caps, if necessary.

Variations

Omit the celery and onion and add ¾ cup (175 mL) finely diced eggplant.

Cook ¼ cup (60 mL) basmati rice, red quinoa or barley separately, then add to the soup with the mushrooms. Quinoa and rice take 20 to 25 minutes to cook. Barley takes 25 minutes if presoaked overnight, or 45 minutes if not soaked. (*Note:* Barley contains gluten.)

Nutrients per serving	
Calories	63
Total Fat Saturated Fat Omega-3	0.5 g 0.2 g 0.0 g
Carbohydrate	13 g
Fiber	3.0 g (12% DV)
Protein	2 g
Biotin	3 mcg (10% DV)
Vitamin C	16 mg (27% DV)
Iron	0.6 mg (3% DV)
Magnesium	28 mg (7% DV)
Zinc	0.5 mg (3% DV)

Chicken and Barley Soup

¼ cup	barley, rinsed, or basmati rice	60 mL
2	boneless skinless chicken thighs	2
	Juice of ½ lemon	
3	thin slices eggplant, finely diced	3
1	red onion (or 3 stalks celery), finely chopped	1
1	carrot, diced	1
2 tsp	vegetable bouillon powder	10 mL
1 tsp	grated gingerroot	5 mL
6 cups	water	1.5 L
1 tbsp	finely chopped fresh parsley	15 mL

Makes 3 servings

Here's a delicious country-style chicken soup. Soak the barley overnight to reduce cooking time and increase mineral availability, or skip the soak and simply cook it for longer. Barley contains gluten, so if you are gluten intolerant use basmati rice instead, adding it with the eggplant.

Tip

If you are vegetarian or vegan, simply omit the chicken.

1. Place barley in a small saucepan of water and bring to a boil, then reduce heat and let simmer for 25 minutes if barley is presoaked or 45 minutes if not presoaked. Drain and set aside.

2. Meanwhile, dice chicken and marinate it in lemon juice for at least 10 minutes.

3. Place eggplant, red onion, carrot, bouillon, ginger and water in a stockpot or large saucepan, cover and bring to a boil. Reduce heat to low and simmer for 10 minutes.

4. Add cooked barley, chicken and 1 tsp (5 mL) lemon juice from the marinade. Simmer for 5 minutes or until chicken is no longer pink inside (for tender chicken, don't overcook). Remove from heat and stir in parsley.

Nutrients per serving	
Calories	170
Total Fat	4.4 g
Saturated Fat	1.2 g
Omega-3	0.1 g
Carbohydrate	22 g
Fiber	4.9 g (20% DV)
Protein	12 g
Biotin	3 mcg (10% DV)
Vitamin C	10 mg (17% DV)
Iron	1.2 mg (7% DV)
Magnesium	39 mg (10% DV)
Zinc	1.5 mg (10% DV)

Mediterranean Seafood Soup

For this lovely, flavorsome soup, you can use a firm white fish that is low in mercury (see page 85), salmon or trout, or 14 oz (400 g) good-quality seafood marinara mix (if it does not contain basa or high-mercury fish). The bean sprouts and lemon are important alkalizing ingredients that give this meal acid–alkaline balance.

3	large plum (Roma) tomatoes (whole, must have no cuts)	3
1	large red onion, finely chopped	1
2	garlic cloves, minced	2
1½ tsp	smoked paprika	7 mL
1 tsp	ground cumin	5 mL
3½ cups	boiling water	875 mL
1 tbsp	vegetable bouillon powder	15 mL
6	shrimp, peeled and deveined (see box, opposite)	6
7 oz	skinless white fish fillet, cut into 1-inch (2.5 cm) pieces	210 g
3½ oz	calamari rings (or calamari tube, sliced)	100 g
	Juice of ½ lemon	
½ cup	fresh cilantro leaves, plus extra for garnish	125 mL
½ cup	bean sprouts, washed in water with a splash of vinegar	125 mL

1. Place tomatoes in a small saucepan and cover with water. Bring to a boil, then reduce heat and simmer for 5 minutes or until skins split. Remove tomatoes from saucepan and let cool slightly, then remove and discard skins and hard core. Slice tomatoes and mash the soft flesh until runny.

2. Heat a large saucepan over medium heat. Add red onion and 1 tbsp (15 mL) water; sauté for 3 to 4 minutes or until onion is softened. Reduce heat and add garlic, paprika and cumin; sauté for 30 seconds or until aromatic (be careful not to burn the spices).

3. Add mashed tomato, boiling water and bouillon; increase heat and bring to a boil. Reduce heat and simmer for 5 minutes.

Nutrients per serving	
Calories	289
Total Fat	9.4 g
Saturated Fat	2.1 g
Omega-3	0.6 g
Carbohydrate	19 g
Fiber	3.7 g (15% DV)
Protein	35 g
Biotin	6 mcg (20% DV)
Vitamin C	30 mg (50% DV)
Iron	2.3 mg (13% DV)
Magnesium	96 mg (24% DV)
Zinc	2.6 mg (17% DV)

Tips

The tomato skins won't split in step 1 if the tomatoes have been cut, so make sure the skins are intact before adding them to the water.

Raw shrimp are often treated with a sulfite preservative, so avoid them if you are sensitive to sulfites. However, some *cooked* shrimp are sulfite-free; your local fishmonger can advise on which ones these are.

Variations

Add ¼ cup (60 mL) cooked quinoa (red or white) or basmati rice to the soup.

Zest the lemon before juicing it and add the zest to the soup, or add ½ tsp (2 mL) grated gingerroot.

4. Add shrimp, fish and calamari; simmer for 5 minutes or until shrimp are pink and opaque and fish is opaque and flakes easily when tested with a fork.

5. Remove from heat and stir in 1 tbsp (15 mL) lemon juice (or more, if desired) and cilantro. Top with bean sprouts. Garnish with extra cilantro.

How to Peel and Devein a Shrimp

1. If necessary, remove the head by digging your thumbnail under one side.

2. Dig your thumbnail into the underbelly and unwrap the shell from the meat. Repeat until you reach the tail.

3. If desired, dig your thumbnail into the underside of the tail and split it, then gently remove the tail. (Some people like to leave the tail on for presentation and then remove them at the dinner table — it's up to you.)

4. Use a knife to make a very shallow cut along one-third of the back, then pull out the "vein." Rinse the shrimp, if necessary.

Use shrimp in Mediterranean Seafood Soup (opposite) or pop them on skewers — you can follow the Oregano Chicken Skewers recipe (page 208).

Guava and Arugula Salad

This tasty salad is rich in fiber, flavonoids and vitamin C. Serve with cooked marinated chicken or Parcel-Baked Fish (page 204).

Tips

If Kumatoes are not available, substitute plum (Roma), vine-ripened or grape tomatoes.

If you can't find small red guavas, substitute ½ large apple guava, 2 fresh figs or ½ cup (125 mL) pomegranate seeds.

Do not refrigerate guava. It tastes ripe and delicious at room temperature.

3 cups	arugula or mixed lettuce	750 mL
2	green onions, green parts chopped diagonally	2
1 tbsp	Halo Dressing (page 224)	15 mL
4	small Kumatoes (see tip, at left), halved	4
2	small red guavas, seeded and sliced	2
½	avocado, sliced	½
½ tsp	black sesame seeds	2 mL

1. Place arugula and green onions in a salad bowl. Add dressing and lightly toss to coat. Top with Kumatoes, guavas and avocado. Sprinkle with sesame seeds.

Nutrients per serving	
Calories	174
Total Fat	10.2 g
Saturated Fat	1.5 g
Omega-3	0.4 g
Carbohydrate	21 g
Fiber	8.8 g (35% DV)
Protein	5 g
Biotin	7 mcg (23% DV)
Vitamin C	155 mg (258% DV)
Iron	1.5 mg (8% DV)
Magnesium	60 mg (15% DV)
Zinc	0.9 mg (6% DV)

Mango and Black Sesame Salad

Makes 2 side-dish servings

Tips

If Kumatoes are not available, substitute plum (Roma), vine-ripened or grape tomatoes.

To tell if an avocado is ripe, gently press on the tip — if it's soft, it's ripe. But if the whole avocado is soft, it may be overripe and starting to bruise.

If you have oily or blemish-prone skin, omit the salad dressing and use a squeeze of fresh lime juice instead.

3 cups	mixed baby salad leaves	750 mL
4	small Kumatoes (see tip, at left), halved	2
1	mango, diced	1
½	avocado, sliced	½
1 tbsp	Halo Dressing (page 224)	15 mL
1 tsp	black sesame seeds	5 mL

1. Arrange salad leaves on a platter and arrange Kumatoes, mango and avocado on top. Drizzle with dressing and sprinkle with sesame seeds.

Nutrients per serving	
Calories	237

Total Fat
  Saturated Fat
  Omega-3
	10.5 g
	1.6 g
	0.5 g

Carbohydrate	37 g
Fiber	8.4 g (34% DV)
Protein	5 g
Biotin	8 mcg (27% DV)
Vitamin C	88 mg (147% DV)
Iron	1.6 mg (9% DV)
Magnesium	57 mg (14% DV)
Zinc	0.9 mg (6% DV)

Beet and Carrot Salad

Makes 4 side-dish servings

Beets are rich in betalain, which boosts the feel-good chemical serotonin in the brain, plus pigmented phytochemicals that protect DNA from damage. Here, they're teamed with the goodness of lemon, apple and carrot.

3	carrots	3
2	large green apples, peeled	2
1	small beet, trimmed and peeled	1
	Juice of ½ lemon	
	Juice of ½ orange (about ¼ cup/60 mL)	
	Handful of pomegranate seeds (or sultana raisins)	
	Black sesame seeds	

1. Using a large grater or a food processor, grate carrots, apples and beet. Transfer to a non-metallic bowl.

2. Add lemon juice, orange juice and pomegranate seeds; toss until well combined. Just before serving, sprinkle with sesame seeds.

Nutrients per serving	
Calories	84

Total Fat
  Saturated Fat
  Omega-3
	0.4 g
	0.1 g
	0.0 g

Carbohydrate	21 g
Fiber	4.1 g (16% DV)
Protein	1 g
Biotin	4 mcg (12% DV)
Vitamin C	19 mg (32% DV)
Iron	0.5 mg (3% DV)
Magnesium	17 mg (4% DV)
Zinc	0.2 mg (1% DV)

Sweet Potato Salad

This is not an old-fashioned potato salad; the sweet potato stays whole while it's baked to perfection. Add some canned tuna or raw almonds for protein and variety, or serve with Oregano Chicken Skewers (page 208). Double the recipe so you have leftovers to enjoy the next day.

Tips

If you have oily or blemish-prone skin, replace the rice bran oil with extra virgin olive oil.

To speed up the cooking time in step 1, cut the sweet potatoes in half lengthwise before baking.

Nutrients per serving	
Calories	321
Total Fat	17.4 g
Saturated Fat	2.7 g
Omega-3	0.2 g
Carbohydrate	41 g
Fiber	12.9 g (52% DV)
Protein	6 g
Biotin	8 mcg (27% DV)
Vitamin C	38 mg (63% DV)
Iron	2.6 mg (14% DV)
Magnesium	83 mg (21% DV)
Zinc	1.3 mg (9% DV)

- **Preheat oven to 350°F (180°C)**
- **Baking sheet, lined with parchment paper**

2	small sweet potatoes	2
1 tsp	lemon juice	5 mL
1 tsp	rice bran oil (see tip, at left)	5 mL
	Sea salt (preferably Celtic)	
1	sprig fresh rosemary or lemon thyme (optional)	1
4	handfuls mixed salad leaves	4
1	lime wedge	1
2	Kumatoes or vine-ripened tomatoes, sliced	2
	Avocado and Thyme Dip (page 229)	
	Black sesame seeds (optional)	

1. Place sweet potatoes on prepared baking sheet. Combine lemon juice and oil; rub or brush onto sweet potatoes. Sprinkle with salt and top with rosemary (if using). Bake for 30 minutes or until potatoes are easily pierced with a fork.

2. Halve sweet potatoes lengthwise and open them like a hot dog bun. Place on serving plates and arrange salad leaves to the side. Squeeze a little lime juice over both potato and salad. Top sweet potatoes with Kumatoes and dollop salad with dip. Sprinkle with sesame seeds, if desired.

Variation

Use Anchovy and Mustard Dressing (page 223) or Beet and Almond Dip (page 230) instead of the Avocado and Thyme Dip.

Quinoa and Pomegranate Salad

Makes 2 main-dish servings (or 5 side-dish servings)

This antioxidant-rich salad is a classic dinner party dish, with a delicate balance of flavors. It is acid–alkaline balanced, and the red quinoa contains anthocyanins and has a lower GI than the white variety.

1 cup	red quinoa, rinsed	250 mL
2 tsp	vegetable bouillon powder	10 mL
2½ cups	water	625 mL
1	large pomegranate	1
¼ tsp	ground cinnamon	1 mL
	Juice of 1 large lime (about 3 tbsp/45 mL)	
1 tsp	extra virgin olive oil	5 mL
½ cup	raw almonds, chopped (see tip, at right)	125 mL
1 cup	fresh mint leaves, finely chopped	250 mL

1. Place quinoa, bouillon and water in a saucepan, cover and bring to a boil. Reduce heat to low and simmer for about 20 minutes or until quinoa is tender.

2. Meanwhile, remove seeds from pomegranate (see instructions, opposite), discarding any discolored seeds. You will need about 1 cup (250 mL) of pomegranate seeds.

3. Drain quinoa, sprinkle with cinnamon and let cool. Stir in lime juice and oil. Add pomegranate seeds, almonds and mint; toss lightly. Add more lime juice to taste, if desired.

Variation

Replace half the mint with cilantro and top the salad with black sesame seeds.

Nutrients per main-dish serving	
Calories	640

Total Fat
  Saturated Fat
  Omega-3
	23.1 g
	2.3 g
	0.4 g

Carbohydrate	94 g
Fiber	18.3 g (73% DV)
Protein	22 g
Biotin	17 mcg (57% DV)
Vitamin C	27 mg (45% DV)
Iron	10.8 mg (60% DV)
Magnesium	292 mg (73% DV)
Zinc	4.5 mg (30% DV)

Tips

This recipe does not work with black quinoa, which does not soak up liquid well. If you cannot find red quinoa, use white quinoa, which takes 15 to 20 minutes to cook.

If you have oily or blemish-prone skin, omit the almonds or use lightly toasted pine nuts instead.

How to Choose and Seed a Pomegranate

When shopping for a pomegranate, choose a heavy one that has firm, unwrinkled skin with no decaying or soft patches. The easiest way to seed a pomegranate involves submerging it in water — the seeds sink to the bottom, while the white pith floats to the top. Here's how to do it:

1. Place the pomegranate in a bowl of water. Using a sharp knife, cut the top off the pomegranate. You can do this in one long, shallow cut about $1/4$ inch (0.5 cm) deep, following the outer ridge at the top, or in four cuts, like you are creating a square lid.

2. Lift the top off the pomegranate, remove any seeds attached to the top and place them in the water.

3. Note the wedge formations inside the pomegranate caused by the white pith. Make shallow cuts into the skin of the pomegranate along the natural wedge lines — there will be about five wedges, depending on the size of your pomegranate.

4. Break the wedges apart and, keeping them in the water, gently remove the seeds. Throw out as much pith as possible and let the rest float to the top.

5. Scoop out the floating pith and discard any damaged, discolored or whitish seeds. Strain the remaining seeds and drain well.

Tip: Be sure to make shallow cuts into the skin, so you don't damage the seeds.

Mixed Salad Wrap

Makes 1 wrap

Here's a healthy wrap that's rich in anthocyanins from the purple lettuce leaves and Kumatoes. It's quite a large wrap, but if you have a healthy appetite, double the recipe.

Tips

To tell if an avocado is ripe, gently press on the tip — if it's soft, it's ripe. But if the whole avocado is soft, it may be overripe and starting to bruise.

If Kumatoes are not available, substitute plum (Roma), vine-ripened or grape tomatoes.

¼	large avocado	¼
1 tsp	freshly squeezed lemon juice	5 mL
1	Spelt Flatbread (page 214)	1
4	slices roasted sweet potato (optional)	4
1	small green onion, chopped	1
1 cup	mixed salad leaves	250 mL
1½ oz	drained canned chunky tuna or Hummus Dip (page 231)	45 g

Optional Toppings

2	Kumatoes (see tip, at left), chopped	2
	Chopped fresh cilantro	
½	carrot, grated	½

1. Mash the avocado and stir in lemon juice. Spread avocado over flatbread. Arrange sweet potato, green onion, salad leaves and tuna in a strip up the center. Add topping as desired, then roll up flatbread.

How to Roast a Sweet Potato

1	sweet potato	1
½ tsp	rice bran oil or extra virgin olive oil	2 mL
	Squeeze of lemon juice	

1. Preheat oven to 350°F (180°C) and line a baking sheet with parchment paper. Slice sweet potato in half lengthwise. Combine oil and lemon juice; rub or brush onto all surfaces of sweet potato. Bake for 30 minutes or until tender all the way through.

Tip: Roast extra sweet potatoes for use in Mixed Salad Wrap (above) or on pizza.

Nutrients per wrap	
Calories	595
Total Fat	34.6 g
Saturated Fat	5.3 g
Omega-3	0.5 g
Carbohydrate	58 g
Fiber	20.0 g (80% DV)
Protein	24 g
Biotin	8 mcg (27% DV)
Vitamin C	26 mg (43% DV)
Iron	4.6 mg (26% DV)
Magnesium	151 mg (38% DV)
Zinc	3.5 mg (23% DV)

Shiitake Vegetable Casserole

Makes 2 servings

This soupy vegetarian casserole is rich in antioxidants, including selenium and vitamins C, D and E. Shiitake mushrooms are well known for their anti-tumor properties and for lowering blood pressure, strengthening the immune system against viruses and improving liver function, which is essential for healthy skin. If you don't like mushrooms, replace them with ½ cup (125 mL) finely diced eggplant, which is rich in skin-protective anthocyanins.

- **Preheat oven to 350°F (180°C)**
- **Large casserole dish with lid**

2 cups	chopped cauliflower	500 mL
½ cup	sliced shiitake mushroom caps	125 mL
½ cup	finely diced red cabbage	125 mL
1 tbsp	brown rice flour	15 mL
¼ cup	cool water	60 mL
2	cloves garlic, minced	2
1 tbsp	vegetable bouillon powder	15 mL
2½ cups	boiling water	625 mL
	Sprinkle of dried oregano or fresh lemon thyme	
	Sprinkle of ground cinnamon	
¼ cup	fresh parsley leaves, finely chopped	60 mL

1. Place cauliflower, mushrooms and cabbage in casserole dish. Set aside.

2. In a large bowl, combine flour and cool water until smooth. Stir in garlic, bouillon and boiling water. Pour over vegetables and sprinkle with oregano and cinnamon.

3. Cover and bake in preheated oven for 15 minutes or until vegetables are tender. Stir in parsley.

Nutrients per serving	
Calories	76

Total Fat
  Saturated Fat
  Omega-3
	1.1 g
	0.4 g
	0.0 g

Carbohydrate	14 g
Fiber	3.3 g (13% DV)
Protein	5 g
Biotin	5 mcg (17% DV)
Vitamin C	76 mg (127% DV)
Iron	1.4 mg (8% DV)
Magnesium	37 mg (9% DV)
Zinc	0.7 mg (5% DV)

Eggplant and Cauliflower Curry

This tasty vegetarian curry is rich in cancer-protective flavonoids, enhanced by the addition of black pepper. The curry spices, cauliflower and ginger improve phase II liver detoxification (elimination of chemicals and hormones), boost immunity and promote acid–alkaline balance in the body. The eggplant is rich in collagen-protective anthocyanins.

2	cloves garlic, minced	2
1 tbsp	mild yellow curry powder	15 mL
1 tsp	garam masala	5 mL
½ tsp	ground cinnamon	2 mL
2½ cups	Anti-Aging Broth (page 184)	625 mL
1½ cups	chopped cauliflower	375 mL
1 cup	finely diced eggplant	250 mL
1½ tsp	grated gingerroot	7 mL
½ cup	coconut milk	125 mL
½ cup	basmati rice	125 mL
1 cup	loosely packed fresh cilantro leaves, chopped, plus extra for garnish	250 mL
	Ground black pepper	

1. Heat a large saucepan over low heat. Sauté garlic, curry powder, garam masala and cinnamon for 30 seconds or until fragrant. Add broth, increase heat and bring to a boil. Add cauliflower, eggplant, ginger and coconut milk; reduce heat and simmer, stirring occasionally, for 15 minutes.

2. Meanwhile, in another saucepan, cook rice according to package instructions. Drain.

3. Stir cilantro into curry. Serve curry on a bed of rice. Sprinkle with pepper and garnish with extra cilantro.

Nutrients per serving	
Calories	392

Total Fat
  Saturated Fat
  Omega-3
	15.2 g
	12.9 g
	0.0 g

Carbohydrate	60 g
Fiber	8.8 g (35% DV)
Protein	8 g
Biotin	3 mcg (10% DV)
Vitamin C	58 mg (97% DV)
Iron	3.2 mg (18% DV)
Magnesium	69 mg (17% DV)
Zinc	1.2 mg (8% DV)

Winter Spiced Dal

This gluten-free vegetarian meal contains detoxifying spices as well as turmeric, which is rich in anticancer flavonoids. The addition of black pepper enhances the protective effect. Serve with Curry Naan Bread (variation, page 214) if you're not in the midst of the 3-day cleanse.

Variations

If you can't eat onions, substitute 4 stalks of celery, finely diced.

Add 1 tsp (5 mL) grated gingerroot with the garlic, and add a squeeze of lemon juice when garnishing.

Nutrients per serving	
Calories	552
Total Fat	3.9 g
Saturated Fat	0.8 g
Omega-3	0.4 g
Carbohydrate	97 g
Fiber	18.1 g (72% DV)
Protein	38 g
Biotin	3 mcg (10% DV)
Vitamin C	10 mg (17% DV)
Iron	12.1 mg (67% DV)
Magnesium	132 mg (33% DV)
Zinc	6.0 mg (40% DV)

1½ cups	dried red lentils	375 mL
	Water	
1	large red onion, finely chopped	1
2	cloves garlic, minced	2
2 tsp	yellow curry powder (mild or medium heat)	10 mL
1 tsp	garam masala	5 mL
½ tsp	ground cinnamon	2 mL
1	2-inch (5 cm) strip of kombu (seaweed)	1
2 tsp	vegetable bouillon powder	10 mL
1 cup	loosely packed fresh cilantro or parsley leaves, chopped	250 mL
	Ground black pepper	

1. In a large bowl, cover lentils with water. Set aside to soak.

2. Heat a large saucepan over medium heat. Add red onion, garlic and 1 tsp (5 mL) water; sauté for 1 minute. Reduce heat to low and stir in the curry powder, garam masala and cinnamon; sauté for 1 minute.

3. Drain lentils and discard any that are discolored. Add lentils, 2 cups (500 mL) water, kombu and bouillon to the saucepan and bring to a boil. Reduce heat and simmer, breaking up kombu and stirring occasionally, for about 20 minutes or until lentils are soft and dal is smooth (it should not be runny or dry; add a touch more water, if necessary).

4. Stir in most of the cilantro and the pepper. Serve garnished with the remaining cilantro.

Sushi Rolls with Black Sesame

Makes 2 servings

Sushi is low GI, low in AGEs and rich in antioxidants and vitamin D. A sushi mat is not essential but makes it much easier to form a perfect roll.

- **Bamboo sushi mat or clean kitchen towel**

1 cup	sushi rice	250 mL
1½ cups	cold water (approx.)	375 mL
1 tbsp	apple cider vinegar	15 mL
6	sheets nori (seaweed)	6
1 tbsp	black sesame seeds	15 mL

Suggested Fillings

5 to 7 oz	sashimi-quality salmon (must be fresh), thinly sliced	150 to 210 g
½	avocado, sliced into thin spears	½
	Red leaf lettuce or mixed lettuce, chopped	
1	small cucumber, sliced into thin spears	1
½	red bell pepper, thinly sliced	½

Suggested Condiments

Wasabi (optional)

Tamari or soy sauce (preferably reduced-sodium)

Pickled ginger

1. Place rice and cold water in a saucepan and bring to a boil. Reduce heat to low, cover and simmer for 15 minutes. Add extra water, if necessary, a little at a time. Turn the heat off but leave the rice on the stovetop for 5 minutes. The rice should absorb all the water and be soft and sticky. Stir in vinegar while rice is hot, then transfer to a bowl and let cool.

Nutrients per 3 sushi rolls (each made with 3 spears of avocado and 3 slices of salmon)	
Calories	578
Total Fat	13.5 g
Saturated Fat	2.1 g
Omega-3	0.6 g
Carbohydrate	89 g
Fiber	8.0 g (32% DV)
Protein	24 g
Biotin	9 mcg (30% DV)
Vitamin C	49 mg (82% DV)
Iron	5.9 mg (33% DV)
Magnesium	90 mg (23% DV)
Zinc	2.4 mg (16% DV)

Variation

Use cooked chicken slices, sliced tofu or drained canned tuna in place of the salmon.

2. Place a nori sheet, shiny side down, on the sushi mat. Place a bowl of water within reach. Spoon some rice onto the nori. Wet your fingers, then firmly pat down the rice to form a thin, even layer, leaving $3/4$ inch (2 cm) of nori uncovered at the end farthest away from you. Sprinkle the rice with $1/2$ tsp (2 mL) black sesame seeds. Add your filling of choice (such as 3 spears of avocado and 3 thin slices of salmon) in a line across the nori, close to the end nearest you.

3. Wet the exposed end of the nori sheet. Starting at the end nearest you, lift the edge of the mat and begin carefully and tightly rolling up the nori around the filling. Use the mat to help you roll the nori into a tight cylinder. Gently squeeze the mat to slightly compact the rice and hold it together. Press the wet edge of the nori to seal the roll; it should stick firmly. Using a very sharp knife dipped in water, cut each roll in half or into 1-inch (2.5 cm) pieces.

4. Repeat steps 2 and 3 with the remaining nori sheets, rice and fillings.

5. In a small bowl, mix a pea-size portion of wasabi (if using) with 1 to 2 tbsp (15 to 30 mL) tamari. Serve alongside sushi. Place some pickled ginger on each plate.

Parcel-Baked Fish

Makes 2 servings

This Thai-style fish dish is rich in omega-3, and the parcel baking method minimizes AGEs during cooking. Serve with steamed greens, such as green beans, broccolini or asparagus.

Tips

Each serving size of fish should be about the size of the palm of your hand. Fish is usually sold in large pieces, so you will probably only need ½ fillet per adult.

If fish develops white clumps on the sides, it is overcooked.

You can use a sprinkling of hot pepper flakes in place of the fresh chile pepper.

Nutrients per serving	
Calories	431

Total Fat
  Saturated Fat
  Omega-3
	22.3 g
	14.1 g
	1.2 g

Carbohydrate	19 g
Fiber	3.5 g (14% DV)
Protein	39 g
Biotin	9 mcg (30% DV)
Vitamin C	6 mg (10% DV)
Iron	2.4 mg (13% DV)
Magnesium	94 mg (24% DV)
Zinc	1.4 mg (9% DV)

- **Preheat oven to 325°F (160°C)**
- **Two 12-inch (30 cm) long sheets of parchment paper**
- **Deep baking dish**

12 oz	boneless skinless salmon or trout fillet, halved lengthwise (or two 6-oz/175 g fillets)	375 g
⅔ cup	Coconut and Lime Marinade (page 218) or marinade of choice	150 mL
1	medium-large sweet potato, peeled and diced	1
¼ cup	soy milk	60 mL
	Freshly ground black pepper (optional)	
1	small red chile pepper, sliced (optional)	1
¼ cup	fresh cilantro leaves	60 mL

1. Place fish in a shallow dish and pour marinade over top. Cover and refrigerate until ready to use.

2. In a small saucepan of boiling water, boil or steam sweet potato for 10 to 15 minutes or until very soft. Drain and return to saucepan. Mash until lump-free, then stir in soy milk and pepper (if using) to make a creamy mash. Keep warm in the saucepan.

3. Place one piece of parchment paper in baking dish and place one piece of fish on it. Fold up the sides so the marinade does not spill when added. Repeat with the other piece of fish. Top each fillet with chile pepper and spoon on 2 tbsp (30 mL) marinade. Close each parcel by sharply folding over the paper ends several times.

Variations

Sprinkle the fish with grated lime zest before baking.

Use another marinade, such as Peach, Thyme and Chile Marinade (page 216).

4. Bake for 10 to 15 minutes, depending on thickness of the fish (slightly undercooking the fish keeps it lovely and tender). If you want to cook the fish longer, keep the parcels open and cook for 2 minutes, then check again.

5. Open the fish parcels and place on plates. Drizzle with a little of the cooked marinade and top with cilantro. Serve with sweet potato mash.

Steamed Fish with Coconut and Lime Marinade

Makes 2 servings

Use any low-mercury fish, such as salmon or trout (see page 85 for the fish lists). Serve with cooked corn on the cob and steamed asparagus and peas.

- **Steamer basket**

2	boneless fish fillets (about 12 oz/375 g)	2
⅔ cup	Coconut and Lime Marinade (page 218)	150 mL
2 to 4	sprigs fresh cilantro	2 to 4

1. Place fish in a shallow dish, pour half of the marinade over top and turn to coat. Remove fish from marinade, discarding marinade, and place in a steamer basket over a saucepan of simmering water. Steam for 5 to 7 minutes or until fish flakes easily when tested with a fork.

2. Meanwhile, in a separate saucepan, heat the remaining marinade over medium-low heat until steaming.

3. Serve fish garnished with cilantro, with the heated marinade as a sauce on the side.

Nutrients per serving	
Calories	363
Total Fat	21.8 g
Saturated Fat	14.1 g
Omega-3	1.2 g
Carbohydrate	5 g
Fiber	1.5 g (8% DV)
Protein	37 g
Biotin	9 mcg (30% DV)
Vitamin C	5 mg (8% DV)
Iron	1.9 mg (11% DV)
Magnesium	73 mg (18% DV)
Zinc	1.1 mg (7% DV)

Moroccan Lemon Chicken

Makes 2 servings

This antioxidant-rich curry has a mild, sweet flavor. The turmeric, lemon and ginger enhance liver detox-ification (elimination of chemicals and hormones), boost immunity and promote acid–alkaline balance in the body.

Tip

Do not marinate the chicken for more than 10 minutes, or the lemon juice will start to "cook" it.

Variations

Use firm tofu or green beans instead of chicken.

Nutrients per serving	
Calories	467
Total Fat	18.1 g
Saturated Fat	3.8 g
Omega-3	0.2 g
Carbohydrate	52 g
Fiber	5.8 g (23% DV)
Protein	26 g
Biotin	2 mcg (7% DV)
Vitamin C	27 mg (45% DV)
Iron	2.7 mg (15% DV)
Magnesium	49 mg (12% DV)
Zinc	2.4 mg (16% DV)

3	large boneless skinless chicken thighs, cut into $\frac{1}{2}$-inch (1 cm) pieces	3
1	lemon	1
2 tsp	yellow curry powder (mild or medium heat)	10 mL
2 tsp	garam masala	10 mL
2 tsp	brown rice flour or spelt flour	10 mL
1	large red onion, roughly chopped	1
1 tsp	grated gingerroot	5 mL
3 cups	water	750 mL
2 tsp	vegetable bouillon powder	10 mL
$\frac{1}{2}$ cup	basmati rice	125 mL
$\frac{1}{2}$ cup	Sicilian green olives	125 mL
1 cup	loosely packed fresh cilantro leaves, chopped	250 mL

1. Place chicken in a shallow dish. Juice half of the lemon and pour over chicken (see tip, at left). Cut the remaining lemon into 4 wedges and set aside.

2. Place curry powder, garam masala and rice flour in a sealable bag, seal and shake together. Remove chicken from lemon juice, discarding juice. Add chicken to the bag, seal and shake to coat.

3. Heat a large nonstick saucepan or wok over medium heat. Sauté red onion in a little bit of water until soft. Add chicken and ginger; sauté for 1 minute or until spices are fragrant (do not let them burn). Discard any extra flour mixture.

4. Add water, bouillon and 2 lemon wedges to the pan, cover and bring to a boil. Reduce heat to low and simmer for 10 minutes or until chicken is no longer pink inside.

5. Meanwhile, in a small saucepan of boiling water, cook rice according to package instructions. Drain and set aside.

6. Add olives to the chicken mixture and heat for 1 minute. Remove from heat and stir in most of the cilantro. Serve topped with the remaining cilantro, with a lemon wedge on each plate.

Oregano Chicken Skewers

Makes 2 servings

This fun dish is perfect for chicken but also works well for firm tofu, shrimp, salmon and other fresh fish fillets. Try other marinades, too, such as Peach, Thyme and Chile Marinade (page 216).

- **Six to eight 8-inch (20 cm) bamboo skewers, soaked for 15 minutes**
- **Broiler pan or rimmed baking sheet**
- **Steamer basket**

3	large boneless skinless chicken thighs, cut into cubes	3
⅓ cup	Tamari, Lime and Ginger Marinade (page 219)	75 mL
½ cup	red or white quinoa, rinsed	125 mL
2 tsp	vegetable bouillon powder	10 mL
Pinch	ground cinnamon	Pinch
8	very small Kumatoes or grape tomatoes, halved	8
	Large oregano leaves	
	Sea salt (optional)	
8	asparagus spears, ends trimmed	8
2	large red cabbage leaves	2

1. Place chicken in a shallow dish and pour in marinade. Cover and refrigerate until ready to use.

2. Cook quinoa with bouillon and cinnamon (see box, opposite). Set aside.

3. Preheat broiler, with rack 6 inches (15 cm) from heat.

4. Thread half a Kumato onto each skewer, leaving a 2-inch (5 cm) space at the blunt end. In alternating patterns, thread chicken and oregano leaves onto the skewers (2 chicken pieces to 1 oregano leaf). Finish with another half Kumato. Discard excess marinade. Place skewers on broiler pan and season with salt.

5. Broil for 10 to 15 minutes, turning once, or until chicken is no longer pink inside (check often to make sure chicken does not get overcooked).

Nutrients per serving	
Calories	386
Total Fat	11.7 g
Saturated Fat	2.9 g
Omega-3	0.3 g
Carbohydrate	38 g
Fiber	6.3 g (25% DV)
Protein	33 g
Biotin	4 mcg (13% DV)
Vitamin C	25 mg (42% DV)
Iron	5.9 mg (33% DV)
Magnesium	141 mg (35% DV)
Zinc	4.1 mg (27% DV)

Variation

Use salmon or trout cubes and broil for about 5 minutes. Be careful not to overcook.

6. Meanwhile, place about 1 inch (2.5 cm) of water in a large saucepan and bring to a boil. Place asparagus and cabbage in the steamer basket, then place the basket over the boiling water. Steam vegetables for 2 to 3 minutes.

7. Spoon quinoa into cabbage leaves and place one on each plate, along with asparagus and chicken skewers.

How to Cook Quinoa

Here's how to cook a small side serving of quinoa for 2 people.

$\frac{1}{2}$ cup	red or white quinoa, rinsed	125 mL
2 tsp	vegetable bouillon powder	10 mL
$1\frac{1}{2}$ cups	water	375 mL
Pinch	ground cinnamon	Pinch

1. In a saucepan, combine quinoa, bouillon and water; cover and bring to a boil. Reduce heat to low and simmer for about 20 minutes or until softened (if using red quinoa, you should see plenty of white). Drain and sprinkle with cinnamon.

Tip: The cinnamon will help keep your blood sugar levels steady while you eat.

Steamed Chicken and Mint Meatballs

Makes 28 meatballs

These healthy meatballs are easy to make and taste great with Ginger and Lime Dipping Sauce (page 222). You'll need a food processor to make them quickly and easily. This recipe makes many meatballs, so freeze the leftovers. Serve with salad or steamed green vegetables and quinoa.

- **Food processor**
- **Steamer basket**

½	red onion, roughly chopped	½
1¼ lbs	boneless skinless chicken thighs, roughly chopped	625 g
½ cup	fresh mint leaves	125 mL
½ cup	fresh cilantro leaves	125 mL
1 tsp	mild yellow curry powder	5 mL
1 tsp	tamari (preferably reduced-sodium)	5 mL
	Brown rice flour or whole-grain spelt flour	
	Sea salt (preferably Celtic) and ground black pepper	

1. In food processor, process onion until finely diced. Add chicken and process until minced. Add mint, cilantro, curry powder and tamari; process until ingredients stick together.

2. Cover a large plate with rice flour and season with salt and pepper. Form chicken mixture into 1½-inch (4 cm) balls. Roll meatballs in flour, dusting off excess, and place on another plate. Discard any excess flour.

Nutrients per meatball	
Calories	31
Total Fat	1.5 g
Saturated Fat	0.4 g
Omega-3	0.0 g
Carbohydrate	0 g
Fiber	0.1 g (0% DV)
Protein	4 g
Biotin	0 mcg (0% DV)
Vitamin C	0 mg (0% DV)
Iron	0.2 mg (1% DV)
Magnesium	4 mg (1% DV)
Zinc	0.4 mg (3% DV)

Tips

Each person will eat about 5 meatballs, so freeze any extras (separated by plastic wrap or parchment paper in airtight containers) after step 2 and cook as needed.

Try using leftover cooked meatballs in a Mixed Salad Wrap (page 198).

If steaming vegetables to serve alongside, after cooking the meatballs briefly clean the steamer basket, then steam greens such as peas, asparagus and broccolini for 3 minutes.

3. Place about 2 inches (5 cm) of water in a saucepan and bring to a boil over high heat. Working in batches, place meatballs in the steamer basket, then place the basket over the boiling water. Cover and steam meatballs for 5 to 7 minutes or until no longer pink inside. Transfer steamed meatballs to paper towels to drain.

Lemon Thyme Pizza

Makes 4 servings

These lovely cheese-free pizzas feature chicken and fresh lemon thyme, an aromatic and therapeutic herb that contains antioxidants and has anti-inflammatory, antibacterial and antifungal activity, thanks to thymol. Thyme leaves also protect cell membranes and increase the beneficial fats within. You have two chicken pizzas to choose from.

Tip

Serve these pizzas with a side salad. If serving without an accompaniment, you may need 1½ to 2 pizzas per person.

Nutrients per serving	
Calories	381
Total Fat Saturated Fat Omega-3	12.9 g 2.7 g 0.3 g
Carbohydrate	49 g
Fiber	9.0 g (36% DV)
Protein	21 g
Biotin	1 mcg (3% DV)
Vitamin C	13 mg (22% DV)
Iron	5.3 mg (29% DV)
Magnesium	101 mg (25% DV)
Zinc	3.1 mg (21% DV)

- **Preheat oven to 350°F (180°C)**
- **2 large baking sheets, lined with parchment paper**

Version 1:
Chicken and Tomato

⅓ cup	Anchovy and Mustard Marinade (page 221)	75 mL
3	boneless skinless chicken thighs, sliced	3
4	Spelt Flatbreads (page 214)	4
½ cup	tomato paste	125 mL
2	vine-ripened tomatoes (or 4 Kumatoes), thinly sliced	2
½ cup	fresh lemon thyme sprigs	125 mL

1. Place chicken in a bowl, pour in all but 1 tbsp (15 mL) marinade and toss to coat. In a nonstick skillet, over medium heat, sauté chicken until no longer pink inside (the mustard seeds will pop, so you may need to use a lid). Remove from heat.

2. Place flatbreads on prepared baking sheets. Spread 2 tbsp (30 mL) tomato paste over each flatbread and top with chicken, tomatoes and a generous sprinkle of lemon thyme leaves. Drizzle with the remaining marinade.

3. Bake in preheated oven for 5 minutes or until cooked to your liking. Transfer to a cutting board and cut into slices. Top with plenty of fresh lemon thyme sprigs, about 2 sprigs per slice.

Variations

Use shrimp, vegetables or tofu in place of the chicken.

Use white potato or roasted sweet potato slices, brushed with garlic oil, and steamed asparagus (steamed for only a minute or two).

After cooking, place baby arugula in the middle of the pizzas. Sprinkle with black pepper.

Version 2:
Chicken and Zucchini

¾ cup	Peach, Thyme and Chile Marinade (page 216)	175 mL
3	boneless skinless chicken thighs, sliced	3
4	Spelt Flatbreads (page 214)	4
½ cup	tomato paste	125 mL
1	small zucchini, cut into thin diagonal slices	1
½ cup	fresh lemon thyme sprigs	125 mL

1. Place chicken in a bowl, pour in all but 1 tbsp (15 mL) marinade and toss to coat. In a nonstick skillet, over medium heat, sauté chicken until no longer pink inside. Remove from heat.

2. Place flatbreads on prepared baking sheet. Spread 2 tbsp (30 mL) tomato paste over each flatbread. Arrange zucchini on top and brush with the remaining marinade. Add chicken and a generous sprinkle of lemon thyme leaves.

3. Bake in preheated oven for 5 minutes or until cooked to your liking. Transfer to a cutting board and cut into slices. Top with plenty of fresh lemon thyme sprigs, about 2 sprigs per slice.

Nutrients per 1 of 4 servings	
Calories	366
Total Fat	9.4 g
Saturated Fat	2.2 g
Omega-3	0.2 g
Carbohydrate	55 g
Fiber	10.2 g (42% DV)
Protein	21 g
Biotin	0 mcg (0% DV)
Vitamin C	34 mg (57% DV)
Iron	5.6 mg (31% DV)
Magnesium	108 mg (27% DV)
Zinc	3.1 mg (21% DV)

Spelt Flatbread

Making your own bread is good for the soul. This simple recipe has added cinnamon to keep blood sugar levels steady and to protect against AGE formation during cooking. It's wonderful for making salad wraps and can even be used as a pizza base (see page 212).

Tip

If you have acne or oily skin, use extra virgin olive oil instead of rice bran oil.

Nutrients per wrap	
Calories	216
Total Fat	4.7 g
Saturated Fat	0.9 g
Omega-3	0.1 g
Carbohydrate	39 g
Fiber	6.0 g (24% DV)
Protein	8 g
Biotin	0 mcg (0% DV)
Vitamin C	0 mg (0% DV)
Iron	2.5 mg (14% DV)
Magnesium	75 mg (19% DV)
Zinc	1.8 mg (12% DV)

1¼ cups	plain spelt flour (preferably whole-grain), plus extra	300 mL
1 tsp	finely ground sea salt (preferably Celtic)	5 mL
¼ tsp	ground cinnamon	1 mL
¼ tsp	baking soda	1 mL
⅔ cup	boiling water (approx.)	150 mL
1 tbsp	rice bran oil (see tip, at left)	15 mL

1. In a bowl, combine flour, salt, cinnamon and baking soda (sift together if necessary). Using a knife, stir in boiling water and oil until a dough forms. (Depending on the flour used, you may need more or less water — the dough should not be too stiff or sticky during the kneading process.)

2. Lightly flour a cutting board and turn out the dough. Knead for about 3 minutes or until smooth and elastic, then cut into 4 pieces and roll into balls. Place on a plate, cover with plastic wrap and let rest for 30 minutes on the counter (this is optional; you can cook them right away if necessary).

3. Lightly flour the cutting board again. Using a rolling pin, roll out one of the dough balls into a large, thin circle (make it as thin as possible). Repeat with the remaining dough balls, flouring the board as necessary to prevent sticking.

4. Heat a large nonstick skillet over medium-high heat. Add a flatbread and cook until bubbles appear on top (less than 1 minute). Pop bubbles as they appear so they don't become browned. Turn flatbread over and cook until bubbles appear on the other side. Don't overcook; the bread needs to stay soft. The bread should lighten all over as it's cooking. Repeat until all the flatbreads are cooked.

Variations

Curry Naan Bread: When flouring the cutting board in step 3, sprinkle some curry powder onto the board, mix it with the spelt flour and evenly coat the board. Then roll out your flatbread. Repeat for each flatbread.

Add ¼ tsp (1 mL) ground coriander or curry powder to the dough to increase protection from AGE formation.

Marinades, Sauces and Dressings

Peach, Thyme and Chile Marinade

Makes ¾ cup (175 mL)

This delicate, faintly sweet marinade is rich in antioxidants and complements chicken and fish. Save a couple of tablespoons to use as a decorative sauce for fish or a dipping sauce for shrimp.

- **Food processor or blender**

2	ripe peaches, chopped	2
1 tbsp	fresh oregano leaves	15 mL
1 tbsp	fresh lemon thyme leaves	15 mL
3 tbsp	freshly squeezed lemon juice	45 mL
Pinch	sea salt (preferably Celtic)	Pinch
Pinch	ground black pepper	Pinch
½	small red chile pepper, roughly chopped (or a sprinkle of hot pepper flakes)	½

1. In food processor, process peaches, oregano, lemon thyme, lemon juice, salt and pepper until combined.

2. Add a piece of chile pepper and process until chopped and well combined. Taste and continue adding chile pepper, one piece at a time, until the desired heat is achieved.

Nutrients per 1 tbsp (15 mL)	
Calories	9
Total Fat	0.0 g
Saturated Fat	0.0 g
Omega-3	0.0 g
Carbohydrate	2 g
Fiber	0.4 g (2% DV)
Protein	0 g
Biotin	0 mcg (0% DV)
Vitamin C	6 mg (10% DV)
Iron	0.2 mg (1% DV)
Magnesium	3 mg (1% DV)
Zinc	0.0 mg (0% DV)

Tip

This marinade is best used right before cooking; you do not need to let the meats marinate for hours.

Variations

Add 1 tbsp (15 mL) grated gingerroot.

Use nectarines instead of peaches.

How to Protect Meats from AGE Formation

Marinades that contain acidic ingredients, such as lemon and lime juice, protect protein foods from excessive AGE formation during cooking. They are also wonderful for adding flavor to seafood, fish, meats and tofu.

In addition, lemons and limes are highly alkalizing once in the body, and supply vitamin C for collagen support. They are two of the best fruits for younger skin.

Coconut and Lime Marinade

This Thai-style marinade goes well with tofu or fish in recipes such as Parcel-Baked Fish (page 204).

Tip

This marinade is best used right before cooking; you do not need to let the meats marinate for hours.

Variation

Use a sprinkle of hot pepper flakes in place of the fresh chile pepper, and add 1 tsp (5 mL) minced garlic.

½	small red chile pepper (optional)	½
1 tsp	finely grated gingerroot	5 mL
½ cup	light coconut milk	125 mL
1 tbsp	tamari (preferably reduced-sodium)	15 mL
	Juice of 1 small lime (about 1 tbsp/15 mL)	

1. In a bowl, combine chile pepper (if using), ginger, coconut milk, tamari and lime juice.

Nutrients per 1 tbsp (15 mL)	
Calories	10
Total Fat	0.9 g
Saturated Fat	0.9 g
Omega-3	0.0 g
Carbohydrate	1 g
Fiber	0.3 g (1% DV)
Protein	0 g
Biotin	0 mcg (0% DV)
Vitamin C	1 mg (2% DV)
Iron	0.2 mg (1% DV)
Magnesium	5 mg (1% DV)
Zinc	0.1 mg (1% DV)

Tamari, Lime and Ginger Marinade

Makes about 1/3 cup (75 mL)

Here's another Thai-style marinade that's perfect for meats, fish or tofu. Use on recipes such as Oregano Chicken Skewers (page 208) or Parcel-Baked Fish (page 204).

Tip
This marinade is best used right before cooking; you do not need to let the meats marinate for hours.

Variation
Add 1 tbsp (15 mL) finely chopped fresh cilantro.

1 tsp	freshly grated ginger	5 mL
1/4 cup	tamari (preferably reduced-sodium)	60 mL
1 tbsp	freshly squeezed lime juice	15 mL

1. In a bowl, combine ginger, tamari and lime juice.

Nutrients per 1 tbsp (15 mL)	
Calories	10
Total Fat	0.0 g
Saturated Fat	0.0 g
Omega-3	0.0 g
Carbohydrate	1 g
Fiber	0.1 g (0% DV)
Protein	2 g
Biotin	0 mcg (0% DV)
Vitamin C	1 mg (2% DV)
Iron	0.4 mg (2% DV)
Magnesium	6 mg (2% DV)
Zinc	0.1 mg (1% DV)

Tamari, Lycopene and Lemon Marinade

Tamari, Lycopene and Marinade

> **Makes about 1 cup (250 mL)**

Tomato sauce is rich in lycopene, while lemon supplies vitamin C and reduces AGE formation during cooking. This marinade is perfect for tofu or chicken.

Tips

This marinade is best used right before cooking; you do not need to let the meats marinate for hours.

Store extra marinade in an airtight container in the refrigerator for up to 1 week.

1 tsp	grated gingerroot	5 mL
1 tsp	minced garlic	5 mL
1/3 cup	tomato sauce	75 mL
1/2 cup	tamari (preferably reduced-sodium)	125 mL
1 tbsp	freshly squeezed lemon juice	15 mL
1 tbsp	rice malt syrup or liquid honey	15 mL

1. In a bowl, combine ginger, garlic, tomato sauce, tamari, lemon juice and rice malt syrup.

Nutrients per 1 tbsp (15 mL)	
Calories	11
Total Fat	0.1 g
Saturated Fat	0.0 g
Omega-3	0.0 g
Carbohydrate	2 g
Fiber	0.1 g (0% DV)
Protein	1 g
Biotin	0 mcg (0% DV)
Vitamin C	1 mg (2% DV)
Iron	0.3 mg (2% DV)
Magnesium	4 mg (1% DV)
Zinc	0.1 mg (1% DV)

Anchovy and Mustard Marinade

Makes about 1/3 cup (75 mL)

This savory marinade is ideal for fish or chicken.

Tip

This marinade is best used right before cooking; you do not need to let the meats marinate for hours.

- **Small food processor (optional)**

6	anchovy fillets, drained	6
1/4 cup	soy milk or other non-dairy milk	60 mL
2 tbsp	rice bran oil	30 mL
1 tbsp	whole-grain mustard	15 mL
1 tbsp	freshly squeezed lemon juice	15 mL

1. Place anchovies in a bowl and pour in soy milk; let stand for 1 minute to reduce the fish flavor. Remove fish from milk and rinse. Discard milk.

2. In food processor, process anchovies, oil, mustard and lemon juice until combined. (Or finely slice anchovies and mash with a fork, then combine with the other ingredients, mixing well.)

Nutrients per 1 tbsp (15 mL)	
Calories	66
Total Fat	6.2 g
Saturated Fat	1.2 g
Omega-3	0.2 g
Carbohydrate	1 g
Fiber	0.1 g (0% DV)
Protein	2 g
Biotin	0 mcg (0% DV)
Vitamin C	1 mg (2% DV)
Iron	0.3 mg (2% DV)
Magnesium	7 mg (2% DV)
Zinc	0.2 mg (1% DV)

Ginger and Lime Dipping Sauce

This dipping sauce is ideal with Sushi Rolls with Black Sesame (page 202) or Steamed Chicken and Mint Meatballs (page 210).

½ tsp	grated gingerroot	2 mL
1 tbsp	freshly squeezed lime juice	15 mL
1 tbsp	tamari (preferably reduced-sodium)	15 mL

1. In a small dish, combine ginger, lime juice and tamari.

Nutrients per serving	
Calories	15
Total Fat	0.0 g
Saturated Fat	0.0 g
Omega-3	0.0 g
Carbohydrate	3 g
Fiber	0.2 g (0% DV)
Protein	2 g
Biotin	0 mcg (0% DV)
Vitamin C	5 mg (8% DV)
Iron	0.5 mg (3% DV)
Magnesium	9 mg (2% DV)
Zinc	0.1 mg (1% DV)

Anchovy and Mustard Dressing

Makes about ¼ cup (60 mL)

This flavorful dressing complements Sweet Potato Salad (page 195), or you could make a tasty Niçoise salad with it.

- **Small food processor (optional)**

3	anchovy fillets, drained	3
¼ cup	soy milk or other non-dairy milk	60 mL
2 tsp	extra virgin olive oil	10 mL
2 tsp	whole-grain mustard	10 mL
1 tbsp	apple cider vinegar	15 mL

1. Place anchovies in a bowl and pour in soy milk; let stand for 1 minute to reduce the fish flavor. Remove fish from milk and rinse. Discard milk.

2. In food processor, process anchovies, oil, mustard and vinegar until combined. (Or finely slice anchovies and mash with a fork, then combine with the other ingredients, mixing well.)

Nutrients per 1 tsp (5 mL)	
Calories	12

Total Fat
  Saturated Fat
  Omega-3
	1.0 g
	0.1 g
	0.0 g

Carbohydrate	0 g
Fiber	0.0 g (0% DV)
Protein	1 g
Biotin	0 mcg (0% DV)
Vitamin C	0 mg (0% DV)
Iron	0.1 mg (0% DV)
Magnesium	2 mg (1% DV)
Zinc	0.0 mg (0% DV)

Halo Dressing

Anchovy and

**Makes about
1/2 cup (125 mL)**

Use 1 to 2 teaspoons
(5 to 10 mL) of this
alkalizing dressing per
person on salads or
baked sweet potato
recipes.

Tips

If you have oily or normal
skin, use extra virgin olive
oil; for dry skin, use rice
bran oil.

Flaxseed oil changes the
taste of the dressing, so
adjust the measurements
to suit your palate. Do not
use flaxseed oil on hot
foods, as heat damages
the oil.

1/4 cup	apple cider vinegar (not double-strength)	60 mL
2 tbsp	liquid honey	30 mL
2 tbsp	extra virgin olive oil or rice bran oil (see tip, at left)	30 mL
1 tbsp	flaxseed oil	15 mL

1. Place vinegar, honey, olive oil and flaxseed oil in a jar and shake well. Taste and adjust the flavor as desired (see tip, at left).

Variation

For extra antioxidant power, add 1 tsp (5 mL) minced garlic or a pinch of yellow curry powder.

Nutrients per 1 tsp (5 mL)	
Calories	20
Total Fat	1.6 g
Saturated Fat	0.2 g
Omega-3	0.3 g
Carbohydrate	1 g
Fiber	0.0 g (0% DV)
Protein	0 g
Biotin	0 mcg (0% DV)
Vitamin C	0 mg (0% DV)
Iron	0.0 mg (0% DV)
Magnesium	0 mg (0% DV)
Zinc	0.0 mg (0% DV)

Snacks, Dips and Spreads

Papaya Cups with Lime and Guava

Makes 2 servings

This fresh fruit cup is suitable as a light snack or a healthy dessert.

. . . .

Tip

Do not refrigerate guava; it tastes ripe and delicious at room temperature.

1	papaya, halved and seeds removed	1
1	small red guava (or $\frac{1}{4}$ large apple guava), seeded and sliced	1
	Juice of $\frac{1}{2}$ lime	

1. Fill papaya halves with guava and sprinkle with lime juice.

Variations

Instead of guava, use chopped banana.

For extra antioxidants, sprinkle with black sesame seeds or ground flax seeds (flaxseed meal) and add a few chopped fresh mint leaves.

Nutrients per serving	
Calories	190

Total Fat
  Saturated Fat
  Omega-3
	1.3 g
	0.4 g
	0.2 g

Carbohydrate	48 g
Fiber	8.2 g (33% DV)
Protein	3 g
Biotin	0 mcg (0% DV)
Vitamin C	305 mg (508% DV)
Iron	1.1 mg (6% DV)
Magnesium	89 mg (22% DV)
Zinc	0.4 mg (3% DV)

Lime and Berry Ice Pops

Berries are rich in antioxidants, and coconut water is naturally sweet. With added lime juice, these ice pops are alkalizing and provide vitamin C, for healthy skin.

Tip

Make sure the coconut water you purchase is 100% pure.

- **Ice pop molds**

½ cup	frozen raspberries and/or blueberries	125 mL
2 cups	coconut water (see tip, at left)	250 mL
	Juice of 1 lime	

1. Mash berries, then divide the purée into the base of 6 ice pop molds.

2. Combine coconut water and lime juice; pour over berry purée. Freeze overnight.

Nutrients per serving	
Calories	39

Total Fat
    Saturated Fat
    Omega-3
	0.2 g
	0.1 g
	0.0 g

Carbohydrate	9 g
Fiber	1.8 g (7% DV)
Protein	1 g
Biotin	9 mcg (0% DV)
Vitamin C	8 mg (13% DV)
Iron	0.4 mg (2% DV)
Magnesium	23 mg (6% DV)
Zinc	0.1 mg (1% DV)

Vegetable Platter

This platter of alkalizing vegetables supplies vitamin C, carotenoids and anticancer indoles (an organic compound).

Tip

Protein- and fiber-rich dips to choose from are: Hummus Dip (page 231), Almond Pesto (page 232) or Beet and Almond Dip (page 230). If you choose to use store-bought hummus, make sure it contains no artificial preservatives, raw egg, cheese or other dairy products.

1 cup	chopped broccoli (green or purple)	250 mL
1	small carrot (orange or purple), sliced	1
½	red bell pepper, sliced	½
	Dip of choice (see tip, at left)	

1. Arrange broccoli, carrot and red pepper on a platter. Serve dip alongside.

Variation

Add celery sticks, sliced cucumber, red cabbage and/or mixed sprouts to the platter.

Nutrients per serving	
Calories	37

Total Fat
  Saturated Fat
  Omega-3
	0.3 g
	0.0 g
	0.0 g

Carbohydrate	8 g
Fiber	2.6 g (10% DV)
Protein	2 g
Biotin	2 mcg (7% DV)
Vitamin C	79 mg (132% DV)
Iron	0.5 mg (3% DV)
Magnesium	17 mg (4% DV)
Zinc	0.3 mg (2% DV)

Avocado and Thyme Dip

Makes 2 servings

This lovely alkalizing dip is suitable as a spread for sandwiches or Mixed Salad Wraps (page 198), or for accompanying Sweet Potato Salad (page 195) or a Vegetable Platter (page 228).

Tip

To tell if an avocado is ripe, gently press on the tip — if it's soft, it's ripe. But if the whole avocado is soft, it may be overripe and starting to bruise.

1	ripe avocado	1
2 tsp	freshly squeezed lemon or lime juice	10 mL
2	sprigs lemon thyme, leaves stripped and chopped	2
	Sea salt (preferably Celtic) and cracked black pepper	

1. In a bowl, use a fork to mash avocado, stirring in lemon juice. Stir in lemon thyme leaves. Season to taste with salt and pepper.

Nutrients per serving	
Calories	164

Total Fat
  Saturated Fat
  Omega-3
	14.8 g
	2.2 g
	0.1 g

Carbohydrate	10 g
Fiber	7.1 g (28% DV)
Protein	2 g
Biotin	4 mcg (13% DV)
Vitamin C	16 mg (27% DV)
Iron	1.0 mg (6% DV)
Magnesium	34 mg (9% DV)
Zinc	0.7 mg (5% DV)

Beet and Almond Dip

Makes 1½ cups (375 mL)

This highly alkalizing dip is rich in the potent antioxidant betalain, which gives beets their remarkable color.

Tips

You can soak the almonds for as much as a day to soften them.

Instead of using almonds, use leftover almond meal from making Almond Milk (page 172), adjusting the amount of water as needed (you may need less).

Variation

Add 1 tsp (5 mL) black sesame seeds (for added anthocyanins) and a sprinkle of ground cinnamon.

Nutrients per ¼ cup (60 mL)	
Calories	108
Total Fat	8.6 g
Saturated Fat	0.8 g
Omega-3	0.0 g
Carbohydrate	6 g
Fiber	2.2 g (9% DV)
Protein	4 g
Biotin	8 mcg (27% DV)
Vitamin C	5 mg (8% DV)
Iron	0.9 mg (5% DV)
Magnesium	41 mg (10% DV)
Zinc	0.7 mg (5% DV)

- **Food processor**

1	beet (about 7 oz/210 g), top removed	1
½ cup	whole raw almonds (see tips, at left)	125 mL
1	clove garlic, minced	1
½ tsp	ground cumin	2 mL
½ tsp	sea salt (preferably Celtic)	2 mL
¼ cup	freshly squeezed lemon juice	60 mL
2 to 3 tbsp	water	30 to 45 mL
2 tbsp	tahini	30 mL
1 tsp	apple cider vinegar	5 mL

1. Bring a small pot of water to a boil. Add beet, reduce heat to low and simmer for 30 minutes or until tender.

2. Meanwhile, place almonds in a bowl of water and soak until ready to use.

3. Drain beet and submerge in cold water until chilled. Peel beet and cut into chunks.

4. Drain almonds and transfer to food processor, along with beet, garlic, cumin, salt, lemon juice, 2 tbsp (30 mL) water, tahini and apple cider vinegar. Process until smooth, adding more water, 1 tsp (5 mL) at a time, if necessary.

Hummus Dip

This healthy spread contains calcium and magnesium, and a range of antioxidants, including lemon polyphenols, which can help to balance blood sugar. Serve with vegetable dipping sticks such as red peppers, carrots and celery, or use in place of butter on Spelt Flatbread (page 214).

Tip

If you would like to cook dried chickpeas instead of using canned, use 7 oz (200 g) dried chickpeas and read the Cooking Guide for Legumes (page 86).

- **Food processor**

1	can (14 oz/398 mL) chickpeas, drained and rinsed (see tip, at left)	1
1 tsp	minced garlic	5 mL
1 tsp	ground cumin	5 mL
1/2 tsp	sweet paprika	2 mL
6 tbsp	water	90 mL
1/3 cup	tahini	75 mL
2 tsp	apple cider vinegar	10 mL
1 tsp	liquid honey (optional)	5 mL
	Juice of 1/2 lemon (2 to 3 tbsp/ 30 to 45 mL)	
	Sea salt (preferably Celtic) and ground black pepper (optional)	

1. In food processor, purée chickpeas, garlic, cumin, paprika, water, tahini, vinegar, honey and lemon juice until smooth. Add a small amount of water or extra lemon juice if dip is too thick. Season with salt and pepper, if desired.

2. Use immediately or transfer to an airtight container and refrigerate for up to 1 week.

Nutrients per serving	
Calories	125

Total Fat
  Saturated Fat
  Omega-3
	6.0 g
	0.8 g
	0.1 g

Carbohydrate	15 g
Fiber	2.7 g (11% DV)
Protein	4 g
Biotin	0 mcg (0% DV)
Vitamin C	4 mg (7% DV)
Iron	1.3 mg (7% DV)
Magnesium	26 mg (7% DV)
Zinc	1.0 mg (7% DV)

Almond Pesto

This alkalizing spread is perfect for special occasions. Use it as a dip for the Vegetable Platter (page 228), spread it on Spelt Flatbread (page 214) or add it to Sweet Potato Salad (page 195).

Tip

If possible, soften the almonds by soaking them for up to 1 day before use.

Variation

If almonds give you breakouts, use raw cashews instead (cashews are not alkalizing, but the other ingredients are).

Nutrients per ¼ cup (60 mL)	
Calories	221
Total Fat	20.9 g
Saturated Fat	2.1 g
Omega-3	0.1 g
Carbohydrate	6 g
Fiber	3.1 g (12% DV)
Protein	5 g
Biotin	15 mcg (50% DV)
Vitamin C	7 mg (12% DV)
Iron	1.3 mg (7% DV)
Magnesium	67 mg (17% DV)
Zinc	0.8 mg (5% DV)

- **Food processor**

1	large bunch parsley	1
1 cup	whole raw almonds (see tip, at left)	250 mL
1 tsp	minced garlic (or to taste)	5 mL
¼ cup	water	60 mL
¼ cup	extra virgin olive oil	60 mL
1 tbsp	apple cider vinegar	15 mL
	Sea salt (preferably Celtic)	

1. Cut off bottom half of stems of parsley, wash leaves in a bowl of water and shake off excess water.

2. Place parsley in food processor, along with almonds, garlic, water, oil and vinegar; process until a paste forms. Season to taste with salt.

Banana Carob Spread

Makes 2 to 3 servings

Enjoy this sweet, alkalizing spread on lightly toasted spelt sourdough bread or Spelt Flatbread (page 214).

Tip
Store leftovers in a small jar and use within 2 days.

1	ripe banana, mashed	1
¼	avocado, mashed	¼
1 tsp	carob powder	5 mL

1. In a bowl, combine banana, avocado and carob powder.

Nutrients per 1 of 3 servings	
Calories	63
Total Fat	2.6 g
Saturated Fat	0.4 g
Omega-3	0.0 g
Carbohydrate	11 g
Fiber	2.4 g (10% DV)
Protein	1 g
Biotin	2 mcg (7% DV)
Vitamin C	5 mg (8% DV)
Iron	0.2 mg (1% DV)
Magnesium	16 mg (4% DV)
Zinc	0.2 mg (3% DV)

Resources

Karen Fischer's Websites

www.healthbeforebeauty.com
www.theeczemadiet.com
www.eczemadiet.com.au

Further Reading

The AGE-less Way: Escape America's Over-Eating Epidemic, Helen Vlassara (self-published).
The Eczema Diet: Eczema-Safe Food to Stop the Itch and Prevent Eczema for Life, Karen Fischer (Toronto: Robert Rose).
The Healthy Skin Diet: Your Complete Guide to Beautiful Skin in Only 8 Weeks, Karen Fischer (Toronto: Robert Rose).
Timeless Makeup: A Step-By-Step Guide to Looking Younger, Rae Morris (Sydney, Au: Allen & Unwin).

Supplements and Skin Care

If you choose to change your supplement and skin-care routine, you can get started with the following list of brands. Please note that I do not personally endorse or sell the following skin-care and supplement brands and cannot vouch for the quality and skin-type suitability. Brand formulas may change after the printing of this book, and there may be other brands that are more suited to your skin type and budget. I recommend doing your own additional research. Read the review website and, if possible, test products before buying.

Supplements

Take chromium, calcium citrate, vitamin D, magnesium, and collagen-building nutrients zinc, manganese, silica, copper, vitamin C, and iron.

Skin Care

Please check each website for shipping and availability in your country. Note that some products may also be stocked by your local beautician or available at your local health food shop or department store.

Avalon Organics: www.avalonorganics.com (USA)
Colorescience: www.colorescience.com (USA)
Jurlique: www.jurlique.com (Canada and USA)
La Mav Organic Skin Science (samples available): www.lamav.com (Canada and USA)
100 Percent Pure: www.100percentpure.com (USA)
Synergie and Synergie Minerals: www.synergieminerals.com (Canada and USA)
Yes to Carrots; Yes to Blueberries: www.yestocarrots.com (USA)

Skin-Care Product Review Website

Make-Up Alley: www.makeupalley.com

References

Adebamowo, C.A., et al., 2005, High school dietary dairy intake and teenage acne, *Journal of the American Academy of Dermatology*, vol. 52, no. 2, pp. 360–62.

Babizhayev, M.A., et al., 2012, Skin beautification with oral non-hydrolized versions of carnosine and carcinine: effective therapeutic management and cosmetic skincare solutions against oxidative glycation and free-radical production as a causal mechanism of diabetic complications and skin aging, *Journal of Dermatological Treatment*, vol. 23, no. 5, pp. 345–84.

Baumann, L., 2007, Skin ageing and its treatment, *Journal of Pathology*, vol. 211, no. 2, pp. 241–51.

Baxter, R.A., 2008, Anti-aging properties of resveratrol: review and report of a potent new antioxidant skin care formulation, *Journal of Cosmetic Dermatology*, vol. 7, no. 1, pp. 2–7.

Bernstein, E.F., Underhill, C.B., Hahn, P.J., Brown, D.B., and Uitto, J., 1996, Chronic sun exposure alters both the content and distribution of dermal glycosaminoglycans, *British Journal of Dermatology*, vol. 135, no. 2, pp. 255–62.

Bingham, S.A., Pignatelli, B., Pollock, J.R., et al., 1996, Does increased endogenous formation of N-nitroso compounds in the human colon explain the association between red meat and colon cancer?, *Carcinogenesis*, vol. 17, no. 3, pp. 515–23.

Boelsma, E., et al., 2003, Human skin condition and its associations with nutrient concentrations in serum and diet, *American Journal of Clinical Nutrition*, vol. 77, no. 2, pp. 348–55.

Bolte, G, et al., 2001, Margarine consumption and allergy in children, *American Journal of Respiratory and Critical Care Medicine*, vol. 163, no. 1, pp. 277–79.

Boniface, R., and Robert, A.M., 1996, Effect of anthocyanins on human connective tissue metabolism in the human, *Klinische Monatsblätter für Augenheilkunde*, vol. 209, no. 6, pp. 368–72.

Boor, P., et al., 2009, Regular moderate exercise reduces advanced glycation and ameliorates early diabetic nephropathy in obese Zucker rats, *Metabolism*, vol. 58, no. 11, pp. 1669–77.

Butler, S.T., 2011, Sun hazards in your car, *Skin Cancer Foundation Journal*, vol. XXIX, pp. 36–37.

Chong, E.W., et al., 2009, Red meat and chicken consumption and its association with age-related macular degeneration, *American Journal of Epidemiology*, vol. 169, no. 7, pp. 867–76.

Clark, E., and Scerri, L., 2008, Superficial and medium-depth chemical peels, *Clinics in Dermatology*, vol. 26, no. 2, pp. 209–18.

Colven, R.M., and Pinnell, S.R., 1996, Topical vitamin C in aging, *Clinics in Dermatology*, vol. 14, no. 2, p. 227–34.

Danby, F.W., 2010, Nutrition and aging skin: sugar and glycation, *Clinics in Dermatology*, vol. 28, no. 4, pp. 409–11.

De Spirt, S., et al., 2009, Intervention with flaxseed and borage oil supplements modulates skin condition in women, *British Journal of Nutrition*, vol. 101, no. 3, pp. 440–45.

Dearlove, R.P. et al., 2008, Inhibition of protein glycation by extracts of culinary herbs and spices, *Journal of Medicinal Food*, vol. 11, no. 2, pp. 275–81.

Denda, M., 2000, Skin barrier function as a self-organizing system, *Forma*, vol. 15, no. 3, pp. 227–32.

Denda, M., Hosoi, J., and Asida, Y., 2000, Visual imaging of ion distribution in human epidermis, *Biochemical and Biophysical Research Communications*, vol. 272, no. 1, pp. 134–37.

Draelos, Z.D., Yatskayer, M., Raab, S., and Oresajo, C., 2009, An evaluation of the effect of a topical product containing C-xyloside and blueberry extract on the appearance of type II diabetic skin, *Journal of Cosmetic Dermatology*, vol. 8, no. 2, pp. 147–51.

Emery, C.F., et al., 2005, Exercise accelerates wound healing among healthy older adults: a preliminary investigation, *Journal of Gerontology*, vol. 60, no. 11, pp. 1432–36.

Etcoff, N.L., et al., 2011, Cosmetics as a feature of the extended human phenotype: modulation of the perception of biologically important facial signals, *Public Library of Science*, vol. 6, no. 10, e25656.

Farahpour, M.R., et al., 2011, Wound healing activity of flaxseed *Linum usitatissimum L.* in rats, *African Journal of Pharmacy and Pharmacology*, vol. 5, no. 21, pp. 2386–89.

Fartasch, M., et al., 1997, Mode of action of glycolic acid on human stratum corneum: ultrastructural and functional evaluation of the epidermal barrier, *Archives of Dermatological Research*, vol. 289, no. 7, pp. 404–09.

Fitzpatrick, R.E., and Rostan, E.F., 2002, Double-blind, half-face study comparing topical vitamin C and vehicle for rejuvenation of photodamage, *Dermatologic Surgery*, vol. 28, no. 3, pp. 231–36.

Fossen, T., et al., 1998, Flavonoids from red onion (*Allium cepa*), *Phytochemistry*, vol. 47, no. 2, pp. 281–85.

Freiman, A., et al., 2004, Cutaneous effects of smoking, *Journal of Cutaneous Medicine and Surgery*, vol. 8, no. 6, pp. 415–23.

Fuchs, K.O., et al., 2003, The effects of an estrogen and glycolic acid cream on the facial skin of postmenopausal women: a randomized histologic study, *Cutis*, vol. 71, no. 6, pp. 481–88.

Garg, V.K., et al., 2009, Glycolic acid peels versus salicylic-mandelic acid peels in active acne vulgaris and post-acne scarring and hyperpigmentation: a comparative study, *Dermatologic Surgery*, vol. 35, no. 1, pp. 59–65.

Gil, M.I., et al., 2000, Antioxidant activity of pomegranate juice and its relationship with phenolic composition and processing, *Journal of Agricultural and Food Chemistry*, vol. 48, no. 10, pp. 4581–89.

Gugliucci, A., et al., 2009, Short-term low calorie diet intervention reduces serum advanced glycation end products in healthy overweight or obese adults, *Annals of Nutrition and Metabolism*, vol. 54, no. 3, pp. 197–201.

Gupta, S., and Mukhtar, H., 2002, Chemoprevention of skin cancer: current status and future prospects, *Cancer and Metastasis Reviews*, vol. 21, nos. 3–4, pp. 363–80.

Hall, W.L., et al., 2003, Physiological mechanisms mediating aspartame-induced satiety, *Physiology and Behavior*, vol. 78, nos. 4–5, pp. 557–62.

Hlebowicz, J., et al., 2007, Effect of apple cider vinegar on delayed gastric emptying in patients with type 1 diabetes mellitus: a pilot study, *BMC Gastroenterology*, vol. 7, p. 46.

Hodges, R.E., et al. 1969, Experimental scurvy in man, *American Journal of Clinical Nutrition*, vol. 22, no. 5, pp 535–48.

Huang, C.S., et al., 2011, Antihyperglycemic and antioxidative potential of *Psidium guajava* fruit in streptozotocin-induced diabetic rats, *Food and Chemical Toxicology*, vol. 49, no. 9, pp. 2189–95.

Humbert, P.G., et al., 2003, Topical ascorbic acid on photoaged skin. Clinical, topographical and ultrastructural evaluation: double-blind study vs. placebo, *Experimental Dermatology*, vol. 12, no. 3, pp. 237–44.

Ichihashi, M., et al., 2011, Glycation stress and photo-aging in skin, *Anti-Aging Medicine*, vol. 8, no. 3, pp. 23–29.

Ireland, C., Hormones in milk can be dangerous, *Harvard University Gazette*, 7 Dec 2006.

Jagtap, A.G., and Patil, P.B., 2010, Antihyperglycemic activity and inhibition of advanced glycation end product formation by *Cuminum cyminum* in streptozotocin induced diabetic rats, *Food and Chemical Toxicology*, vol. 48, nos. 8–9, pp. 2030–36.

Johnston, C.S., and Gaas, C.A., 2006, Vinegar: medicinal uses and antiglycemic effect, *Medscape General Medicine*, vol. 8, no. 2, p. 61.

Jugdaohsingh, R., et al., 2002, Dietary silicon intake and absorption, *American Journal of Clinical Nutrition*, vol. 75, no. 5, pp. 887–93.

Kafi, R., et al., 2007, Improvement of naturally aged skin with vitamin A (retinol), *Archives of Dermatology*, vol. 143, no. 5, pp. 606–12.

Kalousová, M., et al., 2004, Advanced glycation end-products in patients with chronic alcohol misuse, *Alcohol and Alcoholism*, vol. 39, no. 4, pp. 316–20.

Kim, H.Y., and Kim, K., 2003, Protein glycation inhibitory and antioxidative activities of some plant extracts in vitro, *Journal of Agricultural and Food Chemistry*, vol. 51, no. 6, pp. 1586–91.

Kim, S.J., and Won, Y.H., 1998, The effect of glycolic acid on cultured human skin fibroblasts: cell proliferative effect and increased collagen synthesis, *Journal of Dermatology*, vol. 25, no. 2, p. 85–89.

Kowalczyk, E., et al., 2003, Anthocyanins in medicine, *Polish Journal of Pharmacology*, vol. 55, no. 5, pp. 699–702.

Kripke, D.F., et al., 2002, Mortality associated with sleep duration and insomnia, *Archives of General Psychiatry*, vol. 59, no. 2, pp. 131–36.

Kuwabara, T., 2010, The changes in optical properties of skin related to carbonylation of proteins in the horny layer, *Proceedings of the 11th Annual Meeting of Japanese Photo-Aging Research Society*, p. 29.

Lee, Y.Y., et al., 2007, Eugenol suppressed the expression of lipopolysaccharide-induced proinflammatory mediators in human macrophages, *Journal of Endodontics*, vol. 33, no. 6, pp. 698–702.

Lewis, S., et al., 2008, Alcohol as a cause of cancer, Cancer Institute NSW Monograph, retrieved 12 August 2009: www.cancerinstitute.org.au/cancer_inst/publications/pdfs/pm–2008–03_alcohol–as–a–cause–of–cancer.pdf

Liu, S., et al., 2003, Is intake of breakfast cereals related to total and cause-specific mortality in men?, *American Journal of Clinical Nutrition*, vol. 77, no. 3, pp. 594–99.

Luevano-Contreras, C., et al., 2010, Dietary advanced glycation end products and aging, *Nutrients*, vol. 2, no. 12, pp. 1247–65.

Lustig, R.H., et al., 2012, Public health: the toxic truth about sugar, *Nature*, vol. 482, no. 7383, pp. 27–29.

Milind, P., and Deepa, K., 2011, Clove: a champion spice, *International Journal of Research in Ayurveda and Pharmacy*, vol. 2, no. 1, pp. 47–54.

Mizutani, K., et al., 2000, Resveratrol inhibits AGEs-induced proliferation and collagen synthesis activity in vascular smooth muscle cells from stroke-prone spontaneously hypertensive rats, *Biochemical and Biophysical Research Communications*, vol. 274, no. 1, pp. 61–67.

Monnier, V.M., et al., 2005, Cross-linking of the extracellular matrix by the maillard reaction in aging and diabetes: an update on "a puzzle nearing resolution," *Annals of the New York Academy of Sciences*, vol. 1043, pp. 533–44.

Muthenna, P., Akileshwari, C., and Reddy, G.B., 2012, Ellagic acid, a new antiglycating agent: its inhibition of N?-(carboxymethyl)lysine, *Biochemical Journal*, vol. 442, no. 1, pp. 221–30.

Nash, R., et al., 2006, Cosmetics: they influence more than Caucasian female facial attractiveness, *Journal of Applied Social Psychology*, vol. 36, no. 2, pp. 493–504.

Neukam, K., et al., 2011, Supplementation of flaxseed oil diminishes skin sensitivity and improves skin barrier function and condition, *Skin Pharmacology and Physiology*, vol. 24, no. 2, pp. 67–74.

Nishad Fathima, N., et al., 2009, Collagen-curcumin interaction — a physico-chemical study, *Journal of Chemical Sciences*, vol. 121, no. 4, pp. 509–14.

Ohshima, H., et al., 2009, Melanin and facial skin fluorescence as markers of yellowish discoloration with aging, *Skin Research and Technology*, vol. 15, no. 4, pp. 496–502.

Palmer, D.M., and Kitchin, J.S., 2010, Oxidative damage, skin aging, antioxidants and a novel antioxidant rating system, *Journal of Drugs in Dermatology*, vol. 9, no. 1, pp. 11–15.

Pan, A., et al., 2012, Red meat consumption and mortality: results from 2 prospective cohort studies, *Archives of Internal Medicine*, vol. 172, no. 7, pp. 555–63.

Peijun, M., et al., 1998, Blocking effect of quercetin on the nonenzymatic glycation of aortic collagen, *Chinese Journal of Diabetes*, vol. 1, no. 6, pp. 34–37.

Pepper, E.D., et al., 2010, Antiglycation effects of carnosine and other compounds on the long-term survival of *Escherichia coli*, *Applied and Environmental Microbiology*, vol. 76, no. 24, pp. 7925–30.

Perez-Vicente, A., et al., 2002, In vitro gastrointestinal digestion study of pomegranate juice phenolic compounds, anthocyanins, and vitamin C, *Journal of Agricultural and Food Chemistry*, vol. 50, no. 8, pp. 2308–12.

Popovich, D., et al., 2009, Scurvy: forgotten but definitely not gone, *Journal of Pediatric Health Care*, vol. 23, no. 6, pp. 405–15.

Purba, M., et al., 2001, Skin wrinkling: can food make a difference? *Journal of the American College of Nutrition*, vol. 20, no. 1, pp. 71–80.

Ramful, D., et al., 2010, Citrus fruit extracts reduce advanced glycation end products (AGEs)- and H2O2-induced oxidative stress in human adipocytes, *Journal of Agricultural and Food Chemistry*, vol. 58, pp. 11119–29.

Ranasinghe, P., et al., 2012, Effects of *Cinnamomum zeylanicum* (Ceylon cinnamon) on blood glucose and lipids in diabetic and healthy rat model, *Pharmacognosy Research*, vol. 4, no. 2, pp. 73–79.

Ray, R.C., et al., 2011, Anti-oxidant properties and other functional attributes of tomato: an overview, *International Journal of Food and Fermentation Technology*, vol. 1, no. 2, pp. 139–48.

Saavedra, J.M., Harris, G.D., and Finberg, L., 1991, Capillary refilling (skin turgor) in the assessment of dehydration, *American Journal of Diseases of Children*, vol. 145, no. 3, pp. 296–98.

Sajithlal, G.B., et al., 1998, Effect of curcumin on the advanced glycation and cross-linking of collagen in diabetic rats, *Biochemical Pharmacology*, vol. 56, no. 12, pp. 1607–14.

Sarifakioğlu, N., et al., 2004, A new phenomenon: "sleep lines" on the face, *Scandinavian Journal of Plastic and Reconstructive Surgery and Hand Surgery*, vol. 38, no. 4, pp. 244–47.

Sarin, C.L., Austin, J.C., and Nickel, W.O., 1974, Effects of smoking on digital blood flow velocity, *Journal of the American Medical Association*, vol. 229, no. 10, pp. 1327–28, in Vander Straten M., et al, 2001, Tobacco use and skin disease, *Southern Medical Journal*, vol. 94, no. 6, pp. 621–34.

Sausenthaler, S., et al., 2006, Margarine and butter consumption, eczema and allergic sensitization in children. The LISA birth cohort study, *Pediatric Allergy and Immunology*, vol. 17, no. 2, pp. 85–93.

Schlueter, A.K., and Johnston, C.S., 2011, Vitamin C: overview and update, *Journal of Evidence-Based Complementary & Alternative Medicine*, vol. 16, no. 1, pp. 49–57.

Shanmugam, K. R., et al., 2011, Neuroprotective effect of ginger on anti-oxidant enzymes in streptozotocin-induced diabetic rats, *Food and Chemical Toxicology*, vol. 49, no. 4, pp. 893–97.

Shon, M.Y., et al., 2004, Antimutagenic, antioxidant and free radical scavenging activity of ethyl acetate extracts from white, yellow and red onions, *Food and Chemical Toxicology*, vol. 42, no. 4, pp. 659–66.

Sies, H., and Stahl, W., 2004, Nutritional protection against skin damage from sunlight, *Annual Review of Nutrition*, vol. 24, pp. 173–200.

Stanton, R., 2007, *Complete Book of Food and Nutrition*, Cammeray, Au: Simon & Schuster.

Sumino, H., et al., 2004, Effects of aging, menopause, and hormone replacement on forearm skin elasticity in women, *Journal of the American Geriatrics Society*, vol. 52, no. 6, pp. 945–49.

Tang, S.Y., et al., 2007, Effects of non-enzymatic glycation on cancellous bone fragility, *Bone*, vol. 40, no. 4, pp. 1144–51.

Thaipong, K., et al., 2006, Comparison of ABTS, DPPH, FRAP, and ORAC assays for estimating antioxidant activity from guava fruit extracts, *Journal of Food Composition and Analysis*, vol. 19, nos. 6–7, pp. 669–75.

Thirunavukkarasu, V., et al., 2005, Lipoic acid prevents collagen abnormalities in tail tendon of high-fructose-fed rats, *Diabetes, Obesity and Metabolism*, vol. 7, no. 3, pp. 294–97.

Tickner, F.J., and Medvei, V.C., 1958, Scurvy and the health of European crews in the Indian Ocean in the seventeenth century, *Medical History*, vol. 2, no. 1, pp. 36–46.

Umadevi, S., et al., 2012, Studies on the cardio protective role of gallic acid against AGE-induced cell proliferation and oxidative stress in H9C2 (2-1) cells, *Cardiovascular Toxicology*, vol. 12, no. 4, pp. 304–11.

Uribarri, J., and Tuttle, K.R., 2006, Advanced glycation end products and nephrotoxicity of high-protein diets, *Clinical Journal of the American Society of Nephrology*, vol. 1, no. 6, pp. 1293–99.

Uribarri, J., et al., 2010, Advanced glycation end products in foods and a practical guide to their reduction in the diet, *Journal of the American Dietetic Association*, vol. 110, no. 6, pp. 911–16.

Vander Straten, M., et al., 2001, Tobacco use and skin disease, *Southern Medical Journal*, vol. 94, no. 6, pp. 621–34.

Verdier-Sévrain, S., et al., 2006, Biology of estrogens in skin: implications for skin aging, *Experimental Dermatology*, vol. 15, no. 2, pp. 83–94.

Vinson, J.A., and Howard, H.B., 1996, Inhibition of protein glycation and advanced glycation end products by ascorbic acid and other vitamins and nutrients, *Journal of Nutritional Biochemistry*, vol. 7, no. 12, pp. 659–63.

Vlassara, H., et al., 2009, Protection against loss of innate defenses in adulthood by low advanced glycation end products (AGE) intake: role of the anti-inflammatory AGE receptor-1, *Journal of Clinical Endocrinology & Metabolism*, vol. 94, no. 11, pp. 4483–91.

Voelkle, M.C., et al., 2012, Let me guess how old you are: effects of age, gender, and facial expression on perceptions of age, *Psychology and Aging*, vol. 27, no. 2, pp. 265–77.

Wei, W., et al., 2011, Phytochemicals from berries and grapes inhibited the formation of advanced glycation end-products by scavenging reactive carbonyls, *Food Research International*, vol. 44, no. 9, pp. 2666–73.

Wu, C.H., and Yen, G.C., 2005, Inhibitory effect of naturally occurring flavonoids on the formation of advanced glycation end products, *Journal of Agricultural and Food Chemistry*, vol. 53, no. 8, pp. 3167–73.

Wu, J.-W., et al., 2009, Inhibitory effects of guava (*Psidium guajava* L.) leaf extracts and its active compounds on the glycation process of protein, *Food Chemistry*, vol. 113, no. 1, pp. 78–84.

AGE Food List

Adapted from Table 1 in Uribarri, J., et al., 2010, Advanced glycation end products in foods and a practical guide to their reduction in the diet, *Journal of the American Dietetic Association*, vol. 110, no. 6, pp. 911–16.

Acknowledgments

· ·

The ever-growing supply of science and nutritional biochemistry information has helped me to write this book and to look after my own skin. So I thank the researchers, scientists, and doctors who make their research available to others, and a special thank you to Dr. Jaime Uribarri, professor of medicine at the Mount Sinai School of Medicine in New York, for kindly answering my questions about AGEs. I'd also like to thank the skin-care companies who help us to turn back time. It all helps!

Intuition is valuable, too, and that brought me to Selwa Anthony, the writer's agent, who I thank for helping to make my dream job become a reality. I'm lucky to have my children and they are often the first to test my recipes (in the early experimental stages — sorry and thank you!). And I'm grateful for the love and support from my mom and dad.

And to you — thank you for reading and for striving for better health. May you have younger and more beautiful skin very soon.

Warm wishes,
Karen

Library and Archives Canada Cataloguing in Publication

Fischer, Karen, 1972-
[Younger skin in 28 days]
    28 days to younger skin : the diet program for beautiful skin
including more than 50 recipes / Karen Fischer.

Includes index.
Originally published: Wollombi, N.S.W. : Exisle Publishing Pty Ltd, 2013,
under title: Younger skin in 28 days.
ISBN 978-0-7788-0480-2 (pbk.)

    1. Skin—Care and hygiene. 2. Skin—Diseases—Diet therapy—Recipes.
3. Skin—Aging—Prevention. 4. Cookbooks. I. Title. II. Title: Twenty-eight
days to younger skin.

RL87.F573 2014   646.7'26   C2013-908432-0

Index

Cucumber and Mint Juice, 176
Eggplant and Cauliflower Curry, 200
Ginger and Lime Dipping Sauce, 222
Lemon and Ginger Tea, 181
Moroccan Lemon Chicken, 207
Peach, Thyme and Chile Marinade
(variation), 216
Tamari, Lime and Ginger Marinade,
219
Tamari, Lycopene and Lemon
Marinade, 220
Winter Spiced Dal (variation), 201
glucosamine, 23
glucose, 44
glucosepane, 31
gluten intolerance, 82, 91
glycation, 28, 33. *See also* AGEs
glycemic index (GI), 45
foods low in, 44, 45
glycine, 106
glycolic acid. *See* AHAs; BHA
glycosaminoglycans (GAGs), 22, 25, 46
grains, 81–83. *See also specific grains*
and AGEs, 57
alkalizing and acidifying, 78
as healthy choice, 43, 44
grapefruit, 139
greens, 65–67
Green Glow Juice, 177
Guava and Arugula Salad, 192
Lemon Thyme Pizza (variation), 212
Mango and Black Sesame Salad, 193
Mixed Salad Wrap, 198
Purple Carrot Juice (tip), 178
Scrambled Eggs with Watercress, 171
Sushi Rolls with Black Sesame, 202
Sweet Potato Salad, 195
Watercress Soup, 186
Green Water, 182
guava (red), 70
Guava and Arugula Salad, 192
Papaya Cups with Lime and Guava,
226

H

Halo Dressing, 224
hands, 129, 142
hats, 46, 47, 142, 157

heart disease, 48
herbal teas, 63
herbs and spices, 33. *See also specific*
herbs and spices
hidradenitis suppurativa, 52
hormones, 25
Hummus Dip, 231
hummus (as ingredient)
Mixed Salad Wrap, 198
Watercress Soup, 186
hyaluronic acid, 22–23, 25
hyperpigmentation, 13, 14, 123

I

infections (skin), 12, 13
iodine deficiency, 109
iron, 105, 106, 109

K

kale
Green Glow Juice, 177
Purple Carrot Juice (tip), 178
keratosis, 12
Kumatoes, 74–75. *See also* tomatoes and
tomato sauce
Guava and Arugula Salad, 192
Mango and Black Sesame Salad, 193
Oregano Chicken Skewers, 208
Sweet Potato Salad, 195

L

lactic acid. *See* AHAs; BHA
lamb, 48
Anti-Aging Broth, 184
laughter, 144
lecithin (soy), 79, 123
Flaxseed Lemon Drink, 175
Moisture Boost Smoothie, 174
legumes, 79, 86–87. *See also* beans;
chickpeas; lentils
lemon, 73
Banana, Lemon and Coconut
Smoothie, 173
Flaxseed Lemon Drink, 175
Lemon and Ginger Tea, 181
Lemon and Mint Tea, 182
Moroccan Lemon Chicken, 207

onions, 69
  Anti-Aging Broth, 184
  Chicken and Barley Soup, 189
  Guava and Arugula Salad, 192
  Mediterranean Seafood Soup, 190
  Moroccan Lemon Chicken, 207
oregano
  Oregano Chicken Skewers, 208
  Peach, Thyme and Chile Marinade, 216
overeating, 60
oxidative stress, 53

P

pallor, 14
papaya
  Moisture Boost Smoothie, 174
  Papaya Cups with Lime and Guava, 226
papaya ointment, 125–26
Parcel-Baked Fish, 204
parsley
  Almond Pesto, 232
  Winter Spiced Dal, 201
Peach, Thyme and Chile Marinade, 216
peas, 87. See also chickpeas
peppers
  Peach, Thyme and Chile Marinade, 216
  Sushi Rolls with Black Sesame, 202
  Vegetable Platter, 228
petroleum jelly, 125–26
phytoestrogens, 90
pigmentation, 14, 21
  excessive, 13, 14, 123
Poached Eggs, Perfect, 169
pomegranate seeds, 68–69
  extracting, 197
  Beet and Carrot Salad, 194
  Guava and Arugula Salad (tip), 192
  Quinoa and Pomegranate Salad, 196
Ponce de Léon, Juan, 6–7
pores (enlarged), 13
pork, 49
potassium, 43, 110
potatoes, 78
  Anti-Aging Broth, 184
  Lemon Thyme Pizza (variation), 212
  Watercress Soup, 186
poultry, 48, 49, 79, 83. See also chicken
primers, 131

protein foods, 83–87
  AGE content, 49
  alkalizing and acidifying, 79
  for collagen formation, 106
  vegetarian substitutes, 103
psoriasis, 14
Purple Carrot Juice, 178

Q

quercetin, 69, 75
questionnaires
  about AGE intake, 36–38
  about nutritional deficiencies, 108–13
quinoa (red), 67
  cooking, 209
  Mediterranean Seafood Soup
    (variation), 190
  Oregano Chicken Skewers, 208
  Quinoa and Pomegranate Salad, 196
  Quinoa Porridge, 168
  Shiitake Vegetable Soup (variation),
    188

R

resveratrol, 119
retinol, 116–17
rice. See also specific rice products (below)
  Chicken and Barley Soup, 189
  Eggplant and Cauliflower Curry, 200
  Mediterranean Seafood Soup
    (variation), 190
  Moroccan Lemon Chicken, 207
  Shiitake Vegetable Soup (variation),
    188
  Sushi Rolls with Black Sesame, 202
rice bran oil, 88
  Anchovy and Mustard Marinade, 221
  Sweet Potato Salad, 195
rice malt syrup, 79, 89, 163
rice milk, 91
rosacea, 14

S

salads, 192–97
Salad Wrap, Mixed, 198
salmon
  Oregano Chicken Skewers (variation),
    208

More Great Books
from Robert Rose

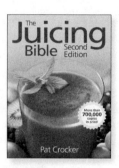

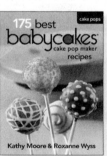

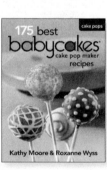

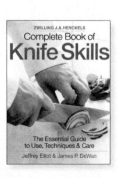

Bestsellers

- The Juicing Bible, Second Edition
  by Pat Crocker
- 175 Best Babycakes™ Cupcake Maker Recipes
  by Kathy Moore and Roxanne Wyss
- 175 Best Babycakes™ Cake Pop Maker Recipes
  by Kathy Moore and Roxanne Wyss
- Eat Raw, Eat Well
  by Douglas McNish
- The Smoothies Bible, Second Edition
  by Pat Crocker
- The Food Substitutions Bible, Second Edition
  by David Joachim
- Zwilling J.A. Henckels Complete Book of Knife Skills
  by Jeffrey Elliot and James P. DeWan

Appliance Bestsellers

- 225 Best Pressure Cooker Recipes
  by Cinda Chavich
- 200 Best Panini Recipes
  by Tiffany Collins
- 125 Best Indoor Grill Recipes
  by Ilana Simon
- The Convection Oven Bible
  by Linda Stephen
- The Fondue Bible
  by Ilana Simon

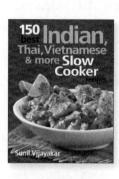

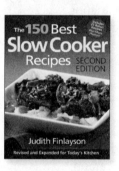

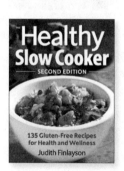

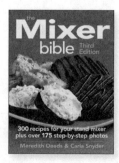

- 150 Best Indian, Thai, Vietnamese & More Slow Cooker Recipes
  by Sunil Vijayakar
- The 150 Best Slow Cooker Recipes, Second Edition
  by Judith Finlayson
- The Vegetarian Slow Cooker
  by Judith Finlayson
- 175 Essential Slow Cooker Classics
  by Judith Finlayson
- The Healthy Slow Cooker, Second Edition
  by Judith Finlayson
- Slow Cooker Winners
  by Donna-Marie Pye
- Canada's Slow Cooker Winners
  by Donna-Marie Pye
- 300 Best Rice Cooker Recipes
  by Katie Chin
- 650 Best Food Processor Recipes
  by George Geary and Judith Finlayson
- The Mixer Bible, Third Edition
  by Meredith Deeds and Carla Snyder
- 300 Best Bread Machine Recipes
  by Donna Washburn and Heather Butt
- 300 Best Canadian Bread Machine Recipes
  by Donna Washburn and Heather Butt

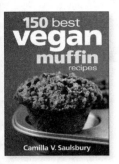

Baking Bestsellers

- 150 Best Gluten-Free Muffin Recipes
  by Camilla V. Saulsbury
- 150 Best Vegan Muffin Recipes
  by Camilla V. Saulsbury
- Piece of Cake!
  by Camilla V. Saulsbury
- 400 Sensational Cookies
  by Linda J. Amendt
- Complete Cake Mix Magic
  by Jill Snider
- 750 Best Muffin Recipes
  by Camilla V. Saulsbury
- 200 Fast & Easy Artisan Breads
  by Judith Fertig

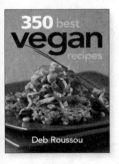

Healthy Cooking Bestsellers

- Canada's Diabetes Meals for Good Health, Second Edition
  by Karen Graham
- Diabetes Meals for Good Health, Second Edition
  by Karen Graham
- 5 Easy Steps to Healthy Cooking
  by Camilla V. Saulsbury
- 350 Best Vegan Recipes
  by Deb Roussou
- The Vegan Cook's Bible
  by Pat Crocker
- The Gluten-Free Baking Book
  by Donna Washburn and Heather Butt

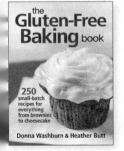

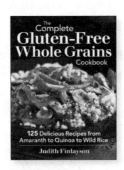

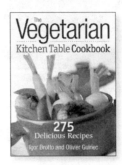

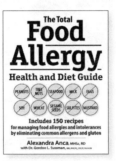

- Complete Gluten-Free Cookbook
  by Donna Washburn and Heather Butt
- 250 Gluten-Free Favorites
  by Donna Washburn and Heather Butt
- Complete Gluten-Free Diet & Nutrition Guide
  by Alexandra Anca and Theresa Santandrea-Cull
- The Complete Gluten-Free Whole Grains Cookbook
  by Judith Finlayson
- The Vegetarian Kitchen Table Cookbook
  by Igor Brotto and Olivier Guiriec

Health Bestsellers

- The Total Food Allergy Health and Diet Guide
  by Alexandra Anca with Dr. Gordon L. Sussman
- The Complete Arthritis Health, Diet Guide & Cookbook
  by Kim Arrey with Dr. Michael R. Starr
- The Essential Cancer Treatment Nutrition Guide & Cookbook
  by Jean LaMantia with Dr. Neil Berinstein
- The Complete Weight-Loss Surgery Guide & Diet Program
  by Sue Ekserci with Dr. Laz Klein
- The PCOS Health & Nutrition Guide
  by Dr. Jillian Stansbury with Dr. Sheila Mitchell

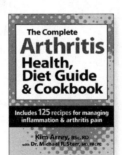

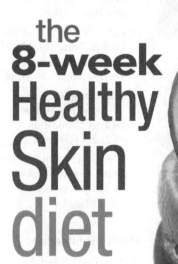